WE 250

T Knowledge and Information Servic

Osteoporosis

HOT TOPICS

Osteoporosis

Michael T. McDermott, M.D.
Director, Endocrinology Practice
University of Colorado Hospital
Aurora, Colorado

Carol Zapalowski, M.D., Ph.D.
Endocrinology Practice
University of Colorado Hospital
Aurora, Colorado

Paul D. Miller, M.D.
Colorado Center for Bone Research
Lakewood, Colorado

HANLEY & BELFUS
An Imprint of Elsevier
St. Louis   London   Philadelphia   Sydney   Toronto

HANLEY & BELFUS
An Imprint of Elsevier

The Curtis Center
170 S Independence Mall W 300E
Philadelphia, Pennsylvania 19106

Osteoporosis Hot Topics   ISBN: 1-56053-628-4

NOTICE

Library of Congress Cataloging-in-Publication Data

McDermott, Michael T.
   Osteoporosis hot topics / Michael T. McDermott, Carol Zapalowski, Paul D. Miller.
    p.; cm.
   Includes index.
   ISBN 1-56053-628-4 (alk. paper)
    1. Osteoporosis. I. Zapalowski, Carol. II. Miller, Paul, 1943- III. Title.
   [DNLM: 1. Osteoporosis. WE 250 M478o 2004]
   RC931.O73M397 2004
   616.7'16—dc22   2004046552

Acquisitions Editor: Linda Belfus
Developmental Editor: Jacqueline Mahon
Publishing Services Manager: Joan Sinclair
Project Manager: Cecelia Bayruns
Designer: Denise Roslonski
Cover Art: Denise Roslonski

Printed in China.

Last digit is the print number: 9 8 7 6 5 4 3 2 1

Contents

DEDICATION

This book is dedicated to our mentors, who have
stimulated our interests and guided our careers;
to our families, who have provided their love
and support; and to our patients, who
are the ultimate reason for our efforts.

Epidemiology of Osteoporosis

chapter

1

Michael T. McDermott, M.D.

Osteoporosis is currently defined as a skeletal disorder characterized by compromised bone strength predisposing to an increased fracture risk.[1] This definition emphasizes that reduced bone strength (bone mass plus bone quality) leads to skeletal fractures and that fractures are the critical events that result in the major morbidity and mortality associated with this condition. Fractures that result from osteoporosis are referred to as fragility fractures, because they occur in the course of normal daily activity or in response to minimal trauma, such as falling from a standing position. The most characteristic fragility fractures are those of the vertebrae, the hip, and the distal radius, but individuals with osteoporosis have an increased susceptibility to all types of skeletal fractures.

The prevalence of osteoporosis by bone densitometry criteria (T score < −2.5; T score is the number of standard deviations the value is above or below the mean value for young normals) among postmenopausal Caucasian women in the United States has been reported to be 10%–18%.[2,3] It has been estimated that approximately 10 million people in the United States have densitometric osteoporosis (T score < −2.5) and another 18 million have osteopenia (−1.0 < T score < −2.5).[4] The number of Americans with low bone mass (28 million) therefore rivals the numbers who have other common disorders such as hypertension (54 million), hypercholesterolemia (52 million), and diabetes mellitus (16–20 million) (Fig. 1-1). Osteoporosis underlies about 1.5 million skeletal fractures each year in the United States, accounting for approximately 700,000 vertebral fractures, 300,000 hip fractures, 250,000 wrist fractures, and 300,000 fractures at other sites annually[4] (Fig. 1-2). In Caucasian women older than 65 years of age, the incidence of hip fractures exceeds that of breast cancer, stroke, and diabetes mellitus.[5] The lifetime hip fracture risk in women exceeds the combined risk of breast cancer, ovarian cancer, and endometrial cancer. One of every two women older than 50 years of age will have at least one osteoporotic fracture during her lifetime.[4]

1

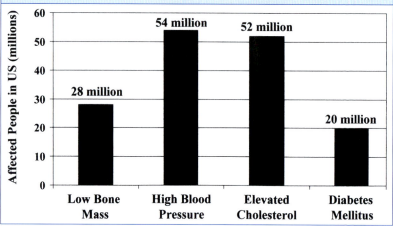

Figure 1-1. The prevalence of low bone mass in the United States is similar to that of other major chronic diseases such as hypertension, hypercholesterolemia, and diabetes mellitus.

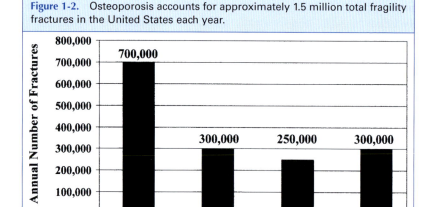

Figure 1-2. Osteoporosis accounts for approximately 1.5 million total fragility fractures in the United States each year.

Osteoporosis has been studied most extensively in Caucasian post-menopausal women, in whom the overall prevalence seems to be the highest. The rates of osteoporosis by densitometry criteria have been reported to be similar or higher in postmenopausal Hispanic and Asian women compared with Caucasian women.[3,6–8] However, the incidence of osteoporotic fractures seems to be lower in these ethnic groups,[6,9–11] probably because of other factors such as higher body weights or shorter hip-axis lengths.[7,12] Native American postmenopausal women seem to have rates of densitometric osteoporosis and osteoporotic fractures that are similar to those seen in Caucasian women.[6,13,14] African-American postmenopausal women, however, have distinctly higher mean bone mineral densities and lower fracture rates than other ethnic groups.[3,6,15]

Approximately 6% of men in the United States (about 1–2 million men) have osteoporosis by bone densitometry criteria (T score < −2.5 with a normal male reference population).[3] A 60-year-old man has a 25% lifetime risk of having an osteoporotic fracture. The lifetime risk for hip fractures in men exceeds that of prostate cancer. Worldwide, approximately 30% of hip fractures occur in men. Compared with women, men have higher mortality rates after hip fractures, approaching 30% in men older than 74 years of age.

The morbidity resulting from vertebral fractures includes pain, kyphosis, loss of height, impaired pulmonary function, and depression. Vertebral fractures are also associated with a moderately increased mortality risk, estimated to be 1%–4% in excess of age-matched normal populations.[16] Wrist fractures also produce significant pain and disability but have not been clearly linked to an excess mortality rate. The greatest morbidity and mortality result from hip fractures, which almost always require hospitalization and can be associated with significant operative and postoperative complications, thromboembolic events, and long-term disability. Approximately 30%–50% of patients are never able to return to normal activities, often requiring assisted walking devices or wheelchairs for mobility, and approximately 20% eventually require placement in long-term care facilities. The mortality rate in the first 6 months after hip fracture exceeds that of the aged-matched normal population by approximately 10%–20%.[6]

The costs of caring for complications of osteoporosis are staggering. In the United States in 1995, osteoporotic fractures accounted for approximately 432,000 hospital admissions, 180,000 nursing home admissions, and 2.5 million physician encounters. The direct cost of caring for these fractures was approximately $13.8 billion. The cost per hip fracture has been estimated to be about $26,000–$37,000.[17] In 1997, there were 40 million postmenopausal women in the United States. This number is expected to double over the next 50 years. Because of this progressive increase in the number of elderly individuals in the population, the costs of managing osteoporotic fractures in the year 2025 are projected to be nearly $64 billion[18] (Fig. 1-3).

Timely diagnosis and effective treatment, discussed in subsequent chapters, can significantly reduce the costs associated with this disease.

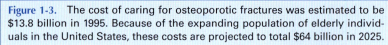

Figure 1-3. The cost of caring for osteoporotic fractures was estimated to be $13.8 billion in 1995. Because of the expanding population of elderly individuals in the United States, these costs are projected to total $64 billion in 2025.

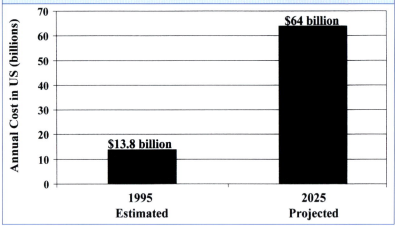

A recent comprehensive analysis indicated that if the number of women older than 65 years of age who have bone mineral density (BMD) testing is increased by just 10% and treatment is initiated when appropriate, the direct costs to Medicare for treating fragility fractures would be reduced by $32.3 million over a 3-year period. Factoring in increased costs of $12.1 million for BMD testing and $4.7 million for adverse events, the net savings for a 10% increase in the current rate of BMD ordering would be $15.5 million over 3 years.[19]

Key Points: Epidemiology of Osteoporosis

- ✍ Osteoporosis is a bone disorder characterized by compromised bone strength predisposing to an increased risk of fragility fractures.
- ✍ Approximately 1.5 million fragility fractures caused by osteoporosis occur each year in the United States.
- ✍ Approximately 10 million Americans have osteoporosis and are therefore at high risk of fragility fractures developing.
- ✍ Osteoporotic fractures are associated with substantial morbidity and a significantly increased mortality risk.
- ✍ In 1995, the cost of caring for people with osteoporotic fractures in the United States was $13.8 billion and is projected to be nearly $64 billion in 2025.

References

1. NIH Consensus Development Conference on Osteoporosis, 2000.
2. Melton LJ III: How many women have osteoporosis now? J Bone Miner Res 10:175–177, 1995.
3. Looker AC, Orwoll ES, Johnston CC Jr, et al: Prevalence of low femoral bone density in older U.S. adults from NHANES III. J Bone Miner Res 12:1761–1768, 1997.
4. Lindsay R: Risk assessment using bone mineral density determination. Osteoporos Int 8(Suppl. 1):S28–31, 1998.
5. Melton LJ III: Epidemiology of hip fractures: implications of the exponential increase with age. Bone 18(Suppl. 3):S121–125, 1996.
6. Siris ES, Miller PD, Barrett-Conner E, et al: Identification and fracture outcomes of undiagnosed low bone mineral density in postmenopausal women. Results from the National Osteoporosis Risk Assessment. JAMA 286:2815–2822, 2001.
7. Villa ML, Marcus R, Ramirez Delay R, et al: Factors contributing to skeletal health of postmenopausal Mexican-American women. J Bone Miner Res 10(8):1233–1242, 1995.
8. Russell-Aulet M, Wang J, Thornton JC, et al: Bone mineral density and mass in cross-sectional study of white and Asian women. J Bone Miner Res 8(5):575–582, 1993.
9. Silverman SL, Madison RE: Decreased incidence of hip fracture in Hispanics, Asians and blacks: California hospital discharge data. Am J Public Health 78(11):1482–1483, 1998.
10. Bauer RL: Ethnic differences in hip fracture: a reduced incidence in Mexican Americans. Am J Epidemiol 127(1):145–149, 1988.
11. Maggi S, Kelsey JL, Litvak J, et al: Incidence of hip fractures in the elderly: a cross-national analysis. Osteoporos Int. 1(4):232–241, 1991.
12. Cummings SR, Cauley JA, Palermo L, et al: Racial differences in hip axis lengths might explain racial differences in rates of hip fracture. Study of Osteoporotic Fractures Research Group. Osteoporos Int 4(4):226–229, 1994.
13. Martin MC, Block JE, Sanchez SD, et al: Menopause without symptoms: the endocrinology of menopause among rural Mayan Indians. Am J Obstet Gynecol 168:1843–1845, 1993.
14. Perry HM, Bernard M, Horowitz M, et al: The effect of aging on bone mineral metabolism and bone mass in Native American women. J Am Geriatr Soc 46:1418–1422, 1998.
15. Farmer ME, White LR, Brody JA, et al: Race and sex differences in hip fracture incidence. Am J Public Health 74(12):1374–1380, 1984.
16. Cooper C, Atkinson EJ, Jacobsen SJ, et al: Population-based study of survival after osteoporotic fractures. Am J Epidemiol 137:1001–1005, 1993.
17. Ray NF, Chan JK, Thamer M, et al: Medical expenditures for the treatment of osteoporotic fractures in the United States in 1995: report from the National Osteoporosis Foundation. J Bone Miner Res. 12(1):24–35, 1997.
18. Cooper C, Campion G, Melton LJ III: Hip fractures in the elderly: a world-wide projection. Osteoporos Int 2:285–289, 1992.
19. King AB, Saag K, Burge RT, et al: The budget impact of current bone mineral density testing rates in the Medicare program. The Annual Meeting of the American College of Rheumatology, New Orleans, LA, October 25–29, 2002, Abstract 1567.

Genetics of Osteoporosis

chapter 2

Carol Zapalowski, M.D., Ph.D.

Osteoporosis is often a multifactorial disease and has a strong genetic component. Bone mass, osteoporosis, and fracture are complex traits subject to the influence of multiple physiologic and environmental factors. Twin studies have shown that genetic factors play a role in determining BMD, skeletal geometry, and bone turnover markers. Other factors that influence bone mineral density and are therefore related to fracture risk are also heritable. These include body mass index, age at menarche, age at menopause, serum parathyroid hormone level, and serum 1,25 dihydroxyvitamin D level.[1] Peak bone mass and rate of bone loss have separately been shown to be under genetic control.[1–4] Sixty to 80% of age-specific variation in BMD at various sites is thought to be genetically determined.[4]

Multiple risk factors exist for fracture; many of these are unrelated to bone strength. A family history of fragility fracture has been shown to be a risk factor for fracture, independent of BMD.[5–7] Site-specific familial fracture risk independent of BMD has also been described.[8–11] Bone size and structure are heritable traits and have been related to fracture risk.[3] Hip-axis length and cortical thickness show genetic variation.[2] The propensity for falling, certainly a complex trait, seems to be a highly heritable trait.[12,13]

Normal genetic variation in complex traits is likely not due to deleterious mutations but to common polymorphisms at different sites. This can lead to changes in gene function or expression, gene-gene interaction, and gene-environment interaction, which may be quite subtle.[3] Although there seems to be heritability of many components of bone strength, nongenetic factors are often of sufficient magnitude to mask the phenotype of these genetic differences.[8] Peak BMD at various sites throughout the skeleton, including spine, hip, and radius, is also genetically determined. The effects of genetics on bone traits are less obvious with age, as environmental factors play a larger role.[8]

In the search for the genes responsible for bone strength, linkage studies in humans and animals have helped to map chromosomal regions that may be involved in the regulation of bone mass and skeletal geometry. Linkage studies involve genotyping large numbers of polymorphic markers throughout the genome and relating them to the inheritance of a phenotype among members of a family. This technique has located and identified genes for many disorders with a clear pattern of Mendelian inheritance. Linkage studies have also been extremely important in finding and characterizing heritable components of complex (i.e. non-Mendelian) traits.[14] Genome-wide linkage studies in humans have identified foci on several chromosomes associated with BMD. To date, the genes that regulate bone mass are only partially characterized.[1]

Candidate Genes Associated with Bone Mineral Density

Another method of searching for the genes responsible for a trait is the evaluation of candidate genes. Candidate genes are chosen on the grounds that they have known or hypothetical effects on a trait, in this case bone metabolism. In these studies, polymorphisms of a particular gene are related to BMD or fracture in population-based or case-control studies. Approximately 20 candidate genes have been shown to be associated with BMD. Most of the recent work has focused on four candidate genes: the vitamin D receptor (VDR), type one (1) collagen alpha (COL1A1 and COL1A2), estrogen receptor alpha (ERα), and transforming growth factor-beta (TGF-β).[1] With candidate gene studies, the demonstration of an association does not necessarily prove cause and effect. The data suggest that multiple genes affect bone mass and fracture risk, each having relatively small effects individually rather than one or two genes with major effects.

The vitamin D receptor is important in regulating calcium absorption, bone cell differentiation, and mineralization. Although the data are conflicting, a meta-analysis suggested that an association exists between VDR polymorphisms and BMD.[15] The association between VDR alleles and BMD may depend on calcium and vitamin D intake, an example of gene-environment interaction.[15,16] Taking into account complex interactions between gene polymorphisms and environmental factors, in this case VDR polymorphisms and calcium and vitamin D intake, may allow better understanding of discordant relationships between genetic traits and gene polymorphisms.

Type 1 collagen is the major bone protein. Type 1 collagen is a triple helix composed of two chains encoded by the COL1A1 gene and one chain encoded by the COL1A2 gene. Deleterious mutations in COL1A1 and COL1A2 have been shown to result in osteogenesis imperfecta (OI).[4,17–19] Osteogenesis imperfecta is a heritable disorder of connective tissue that can be extremely variable in its presentation and severity.

Sometimes referred to as brittle bone disease, in its more severe forms OI results in multiple fractures from birth and skeletal deformity, although it can also present as a much milder form and not be associated with fractures until adulthood, if at all. Many forms of OI also exhibit ligamentous laxity, blue sclerae, defective dentinogenesis, and deafness, all traits associated with the defect in type 1 collagen. Ehlers-Danlos syndrome has also been shown to be associated with an abnormality in type 1 collagen.[20] An association between the COL1A1 alleles and bone density, body mass index, and fracture risk has been shown in population studies as well.[1,17] In the future, the COL1A1 polymorphism may become a useful marker of osteoporotic fracture risk and, together with BMD, may be used to enhance fracture prediction.[21]

The estrogen receptors are in large part responsible for estrogen effects on bone. Estrogen is involved in skeletal growth and the closure of bone epiphyses in adolescents, and the lack of estrogen results in bone loss after menopause. Polymorphisms of the ERα gene have been found to be associated with bone mass in Japanese, American, and European populations.[22] A meta-analysis of polymorphisms suggests that the Xba1, but not the PvuII polymorphisms of the estrogen receptor gene, are associated with both BMD and fracture risk.[23]

Transforming growth factor-beta (TGF-β) is both abundant in bone and an important regulator of bone metabolism. Transforming growth factor-beta 1 is considered a putative regulator of osteoclastic-osteoblastic interaction (coupling). Mutations of this gene result in sclerotic bone dysplasia (Camurati Engelmann disease).[24] Polymorphisms of the TGF-β1 gene have been associated with BMD, osteoporotic fracture, and levels of biochemical markers of bone turnover.[25,26]

A number of smaller studies evaluated other gene polymorphisms. The tumor necrosis factor superfamily 1B candidate gene has been shown in a population-based cohort study to be associated with the regulation of BMD.[27] Corroboration of these data in another study will be required before it can truly be considered a candidate gene. Associations have been shown between polymorphisms at the interleukin-6 gene and biochemical markers of bone turnover and possibly with BMD.[28,29] Insulin-like growth factor-1 has been studied, and the data are conflicting.[30] The ApoE4 allele was related to low bone mass and fractures in different populations.[31,32] This effect may occur by effects on vitamin K transport with subsequent effects on osteocalcin.[1]

Linkage Studies Involving Bone Mineral Density

Linkage studies have identified examples in which low or high BMD is inherited in simple Mendelian fashion. Examples of these include OI (discussed previously) and osteoporosis caused by inactivating mutations in the aromatase gene.[33–35] An extended family has been described in which there is linkage between a genetic locus on chromosome 11 (11q12-13) and very high spinal BMD.[4,36] This is the same region where the autosomally recessive disorder osteoporosis-pseudoglioma syndrome, a syndrome of severe premature osteoporosis often associated with fracture and a bilateral eye disorder that leads to early blindness, was previously mapped.[4] Subsequent studies have revealed that an abnormality of the lipoprotein receptor–related protein 5 (LRP-5) is responsible for both mutations, with an inactivating mutation causing osteoporosis-pseudoglioma syndrome and activating mutations causing the autosomal dominant phenotype of increased BMD.[37,38] Van Wesenbeeck et al performed mutation analysis of the LRP-5 gene in 10 families of isolated patients with different conditions with an increased bone density, including endosteal hyperostosis, Van Buchem disease, autosomal dominant osteosclerosis, and osteopetrosis. They found an association with the LRP-5 gene in all of them, indicating that increased BMD affecting mainly the cortices of long bone and the skull is often caused by mutations in the LRP-5 gene.[39] These data will need corroboration with other studies. As with most single gene mutations leading to disease, these are rare and account for only a small portion of individuals with osteoporosis.

The mechanisms of all the candidate genes described to date and how BMD and fracture risk are directly affected by them is unknown.[1,4] Knowledge about genetic polymorphisms of candidate genes affecting osteoporosis will likely, in the future, allow better prediction of risk for fracture, as well as the ability to target specific dietary or pharmacologic therapies appropriately. The genetic markers of bone fragility may

Key Points: Genetics of Osteoporosis

- ⮞ Twin studies have shown that genetic factors play a role in determining bone mineral density, skeletal geometry, and bone turnover markers.
- ⮞ Sixty to 80% of age-specific variation in bone mineral density at various sites is thought to be genetically determined.
- ⮞ Although there seems to be a heritability of many components of bone strength, nongenetic factors are often of sufficient magnitude to mask the phenotype of these genetic differences. The effects of genetics on bone traits are less obvious with age, as environmental factors play a larger role.

become useful as diagnostic tools, along with bone density measurements to allow identification of those individuals at highest risk for fracture.[1] Ultimately, the understanding of the interactions between genetics and environment on skeletal health will be the cornerstone of new advances in clinical management of osteoporosis and other metabolic bone diseases.

References

1. Ralston SH: Genetic control of susceptibility to osteoporosis. J Clin Endocrinol Metab 87:2460–2466, 2002.
2. Ferrari S, Rizzoli R, Bonjour J-P: Genetic aspects of osteoporosis. Curr Opin Rheumatol 11:294–300, 1999.
3. Peacock M, Turner CH, Econs MJ, et al: Genetics of osteoporosis. Endocrine Rev 23:303–326, 2002.
4. Hobson EE, Ralston SH. Role of genetic factors in the pathophysiology and management of osteoporosis. Clin Endocrinol 54:1–9, 2001.
5. Cummings SR, Nevitt MC, Browner WS, et al: Risk factors for hip fracture in white women. Study of Osteoporotic Fractures Research Group. N Engl J Med 332:767–773, 1995.
6. Torgerson DJ, Campbell MK, Thomas RE, Reid DM. Prediction of perimenopausal fractures by bone mineral density and other risk factors. J Bone Miner Res 11: 293–297, 1996.
7. Deng HW, Chen WM, Recker S, et al: Genetic determination of Colles' fracture and differential bone mass in women with and without Colles' fracture. J Bone Miner Res 15:1243–1252, 2000.
8. Burshell AL, Smith SR: Familial osteoporosis. Osteoporosis 2(2):195–206, 2001.
9. Cummings SR, Nevitt MC, Browner WS, et al: Risk factors for hip fracture in white women. N Engl J Med 332:767–773, 1995.
10. Fox KM, Cummings SR, Powell-Threats K, et al: Family history and risk of osteoporotic fracture. Study of Osteoporotic Fractures Research Group. Osteoporos Int 8: 557–562, 1998.
11. Keen RW, Hart DJ, Arden NK, et al: Family history of appendicular fracture and risk of osteoporosis: a population-based study. Osteoporos Int 10:161–166, 1999.
12. Carmelli D, Kelly-Hayes M, Wolf PA, et al: The contribution of genetic influences to measures of lower-extremity function in older male twins [Journal Article. Twin Study]. J Gerontol, Series A-Biological Sciences & Medical Sciences 55(1): B49–B53, 2000.
13. Wark JD, Hill K, Cassano AM, et al: Genetic effects on falls risk may help explain why fractures run in families: a twin study. Bone 28(Suppl.):S72 (Abstract ORII), 2001.
14. Housman D: Human DNA polymorphisms. N Engl J Med 332:318–320, 1995.
15. Gong G, Stern HS, Cheng SC, et al: The association of bone mineral density with vitamin D receptor gene polymorphisms. Osteoporos Int 9:55–64, 1999.
16. Ferrari S, Rizzoli R, Slosman D, et al: Do dietary calcium and age explain the controversy surrounding the relationship between bone mineral density and vitamin D receptor gene polymorphisms? J Bone Miner Res 13:363–370, 1998.
17. Mann V, Hobson EE, Li B, et al: A COL1A1 Sp1 binding site polymorphism predisposes to osteoporotic fracture by affecting bone density and quality. J Clin Invest 107:899–907, 2001.

18. Johnson MT, Morrison S, Heeger S, et al: A variant of osteogenesis imperfecta type IV with resolving kyphomelia is caused by a novel COL1A2 mutation. J Med Genet 39:128–132, 2002.

19. Cole WG: Advances in osteogenesis imperfecta. Clin Orthop 1:6–16, 2002.

20. Giunta C, Superti-Furga A, Spranger S, et al: B. Ehlers-Danlos syndrome type VII: clinical features and molecular defects. J Bone Joint Surg Am 81(2):225–238, 1999.

21. McGuigan FE, Armbrecht G, Smith R, et al: Prediction of osteoporotic fractures by bone densitometry and COLIA1 genotyping: a prospective, population-based study in men and women. Osteoporos Int 12:91–96, 2001.

22. Becherini L, Gennari L, Masi L, et al: Evidence of a linkage disequilibrium between polymorphisms in the human estrogen receptor [alpha] gene and their relationship to bone mass variation in postmenopausal Italian women. Hum Mol Genet 9:2043–2050, 2000.

23. Ioannidis JP, Stavrou I, Trikalinos TA, et al: ER-alpha Genetics Meta-Analysis. Association of polymorphisms of the estrogen receptor alpha gene with bone mineral density and fracture risk in women: a meta-analysis. J Bone Miner Res 17:2048–2060, 2002.

24. Janssens K, Gershoni-Baruch R, Guanabens N, et al: Mutations in the latency-associated peptide of TGF[beta]-1 cause Camurati-Engelmann disease. Nat Genet 26:19, 2000.

25. Yamada Y, Miyauchi A, Goto J, et al: Association of a polymorphism of the transforming growth factor-[beta]1 gene with genetic susceptibility to osteoporosis in postmenopausal Japanese women. J Bone Miner Res 13:1569–1576, 1998.

26. Langdahl BL, Knudsen JY, Jensen HK, et al: A sequence variation: 713-8delC in the transforming growth factor-[beta] 1 gene has higher prevalence in osteoporotic women than in normal women and is associated with very low bone mass in osteoporotic women and increased bone turnover in both osteoporotic and normal women. Bone 20:289–229, 1997.

27. Albagha O, Tasker P, McGuigan F, et al: Linkage disequilibrium between polymorphisms in the human TNFRSF1B gene and their association with bone mass in perimenopausal women. Hum Mol Genet 11:2289–2295, 2002.

28. Murray RE, McGuigan F, Grant SFA, et al: Polymorphisms of the Interleukin-6 Gene are associated with bone mineral density. Bone 21:89–92, 1997.

29. Ferrari SL, Ahn-Luong L, Garnero P, et al: Two promoter polymorphisms regulating interleukin-6 gene expression are associated with circulating levels of C-reactive protein and markers of bone resorption in postmenopausal women. J Clin Endocrinol Metab 88:255–259, 2003.

30. Rosen CJ, Bilezikian JP: Perplexing polymorphisms: D(i)ps, Sn(i)ps, and trips [editorial]. J Clin Endocrinol Metab 84:4465–4466, 1999.

31. Shiraki M, Shiraki Y, Aoki C, et al: Association of bone mineral density with apolipoprotein E phenotype. J Bone Miner Res 12:1438–1445, 1997.

32. Cauley JA, Zmuda JM, Jaffe K, et al: Apolipoprotein E polymorphism: a new genetic marker of hip fracture risk. The Study of osteoporotic fractures. J Bone Miner Res 14:1175–1181, 1999.

33. Smith EP, Boyd J, Frank GR, et al: Estrogen resistance caused by a mutation in the estrogen-receptor gene in a man. N Engl J Med 331:1056–1061, 1994.

34. Morishima A, Grumbach MM, Simpson ER, et al: Aromatase deficiency in male and female siblings caused by a novel mutation and the physiological role of estrogens. J Clin Endocrinol Metab 80:3689–3698, 1995.

35. Masi L, Becherini L, Gennari L, et al: Polymorphism of the aromatase gene in postmenopausal Italian women: Distribution and correlation with bone mass and fracture risk. J Clin Endocrinol Metab 86:2263–2269, 2001.

36. Johnson ML, Gong G, Kimberling W, et al: Linkage of a gene causing high bone mass to human chromosome 11(11q12-13). Am J Hum Genet 60:1326–1332, 1997.
37. Gong Y, Slee RB, Fukai N, et al: The Osteoporosis-Pseudoglioma Syndrome Collaborative Group. LDL receptor-related protein 5 (LRP5) affects bone accrual and eye development. Cell 107:513–523, 2001.
38. Little RD, Carulli JP, Del Mastro RG, et al: A mutation in the LDL receptor-related protein 5 gene results in the autosomal dominant high-bone-mass trait. Am J Hum Genet 70:11–19, 2002.
39. Van Wesenbeeck L, Cleiren E, Gram J, et al: Six novel missense mutations in the LDL receptor-related protein 5 (LRP5) gene in different conditions with an increased bone density. Am J Hum Genet 72:763–771, 2003.

Risk Factors for Osteoporosis Fractures

chapter

3

Paul D. Miller, M.D.

The gold standard for the diagnosis of osteoporosis or osteopenia by the World Health Organization (WHO) criteria, as well as for fracture risk assessment, has been central dual-energy x-ray absorptiometry (central DXA). The justification for this standard is the knowledge that most of the WHO criteria for diagnosing osteoporosis before a fracture has occurred have been established by central DXA technologies, especially linking the prevalence of WHO osteoporosis (<−2.5) at the hip (16% in the postmenopausal population 50 years of age and older) to the lifetime risk for hip fracture in this same population (16%).[1] Peripheral bone-density technologies cannot be used for the WHO classification, because only the wrist peripheral BMD device (not any other peripheral technology) was used in the database to establish the WHO criteria and was only used in combination with spine and hip central DXA (not isolation, as was the case for hip measurements) for establishing WHO criteria.[2] In addition, T scores derived from all peripheral BMD measuring devices (as well as central DXA spine and wrist devices) are all still derived from their own manufacturer-specific and inconsistent young-normal reference population databases, which may yield different T scores in the same patient at the same skeletal site and, therefore, WHO classification.[3,4]

Central DXA Devices

For WHO diagnosis, central DXA devices are the accepted norm. The best documented application of peripheral bone mass measurement technologies is for fracture risk prediction. The first prospective observation documenting the ability of any BMD technology to predict fracture risk was in 1988, when forearm BMD was shown to predict an increased risk for nonspinal fractures in postmenopausal women.[5] This study was followed by a large meta-analysis, which documented the value that multiple technologies, both peripheral and central, have to predict an increased risk for vertebral, nonvertebral, and hip fracture injury.[6] It has been suggested that the femoral neck is a more robust skeletal site to predict the risk for hip fracture (relative risk/standard deviation [RR/SD] = 2.4) compared with a peripheral device to predict the risk for hip fracture.[7,8] Although this suggestion of equal fracture prediction for hip fracture risk on the basis of central hip BMD measurements is based on the study of osteoporotic fracture (SOF), a head-to-head hip/heel ultrasound device study, hip fracture risk was also equally predictive of hip fracture in the National Osteoporosis Risk Assessment study (NORA) that used wrist or heel DXA with an RR/SD of 2.4/SD reduction from the mean BMD in a non-head-to-head study. In addition, the receiver operating characteristic (ROC) curves of the two peripheral devices used in NORA match the ROC curves seen with femoral neck DXA obtained from SOF. NORA was not a head-to-head comparison with hip DXA (Fig. 3-1).[9,10] Nevertheless, it seems that peripheral device values, if found to be low in the postmenopausal population, are powerful predictors of hip fracture risk in untreated postmenopausal women.

Figure 3-1.   Receiver operating characteristic (ROC) curve of hip fracture prediction by heel single-energy x-ray absorptiometry (SXA) and forearm dual energy x-ray absorptiometry (pDXA) in the National Osteoporosis Risk Assessment (NORA) study. (Data from Miller PD, Siris ES, Barrett-Conner E, et al. Prediction of fracture risk in postmenopausal Caucasian women with peripheral bone densitometry: evidence from the National Osteoporosis Risk Assessment (NORA). J Bone Miner Res 17:2222–2230, 2002.)

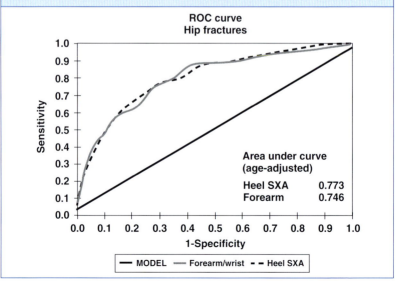

Additional Risk Factors

There are additional risk factors for fracture risk prediction in addition to low central or peripheral BMD. The most important and independent risk factors are prevalent vertebral fractures and increased age. Prevalent vertebral fractures (both the number and severity) are risk factors for both vertebral and hip fractures. The combination of low BMD and prevalent vertebral fractures increases risk above and beyond the increased risk associated with either low BMD or prevalent fractures alone (Fig. 3-2).[11] Increased age also increases risk, even at equivalent levels of BMD (Fig. 3-3).[5] This well-known relationship may be related to several factors: the changes in bone microarchitecture that accompany aging, which render a bone more fragile independent of BMD, and the greater frequency of falling in the elderly population.[12,13] Furthermore, independent risk factors for fracture also contribute to risk. It has been shown that as the number of risk factors increases, so does the risk, again at comparable levels of BMD (Fig. 3-4).[14] The relationship between low BMD and cumulative risk factors is not additive or multiplicative but a mathematical relationship in which the increased risk, as a function of the number of risk factors begins, to plateau as more risk factors are added.[15] The independent factors that add risk to that observed with low BMD alone are shown in Table 3-1.[16] The most

Figure 3-2. The relationship between BMD and prevalent vertebral fractures on the subsequent risk of future vertebral fractures. (Adapted from Ross PD, Davis JW, Epstein RS, et al. Pre-existing fracture and bone mass predict vertebral fracture incidence in women. Ann Intern Med 114:919–923, 1998.)

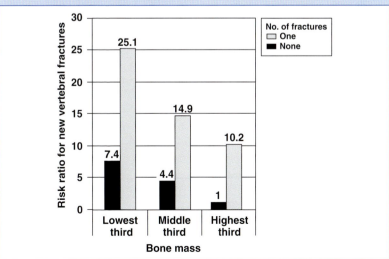

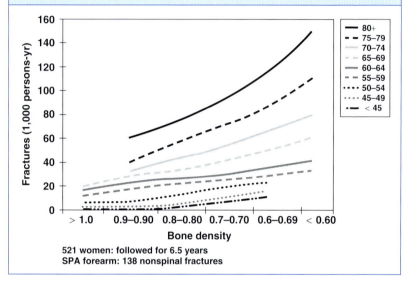

Figure 3-3. Influence of increasing age on risk for fracture at comparable bone mineral content values. (Adapted from Hui SL, Slemenda CW, Johnston CC Jr. Age and bone mass as predictors of fracture in a prospective study, J Clin Invest 81:1804–1809, 1988.)

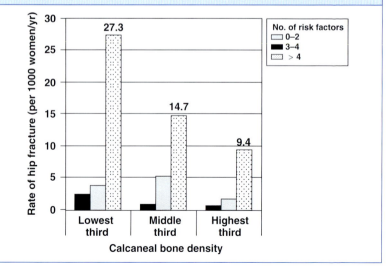

Figure 3-4. Influence of the combination of low BMD and cumulative risk factors on the absolute hip fracture risk in postmenopausal women. (Adapted from Cummings SR, Nevitt MC, Browner WS, et al. Risk factors for hip fracture in white women. N Engl J Med 332:76, 1995.)

Table 3-1.	Independent Risk Factors for Hip Fracture
• Elevated N-telopeptide: 2.0	• Current smoking: 1.2
• Prior fragility fracture: 1.3	• Poor visual acuity: 2.0
• Low body weight: 1.4	• Poor visual depth: 2.0
• Long hip axis: 1.9	• Low gait speed: 1.3
• First-degree relative with fragility fracture: 1.5	• Increase body sway: 1.7
• Maternal history of hip fracture: 1.9	• Poor tandem gait: 1.4
	• Low BMD: 2.7

Data from Kanis JA: Risk factors for hip fracture. Osteoporos Int 11:120, 2000.

important risk factors are low BMD, increased age, prevalent vertebral fractures, maternal history of hip fracture, and low body weight.

Gender and Risk

What about risk prediction in men and women of other ethnic groups? Data from head-to-head trials compare fracture rates in Caucasian men and women; both genders have the same absolute hip fracture risk at the same absolute BMD at the femoral neck; and both Caucasian men and women have the same 10-year absolute hip fracture risk at the same T score when the T score is derived from the female National Health and Nutrition Examination Survery III (NHANES III) reference hip database.[17,18] These head-to-head comparisons, whether based on absolute BMD or on SD scores, would suggest that there may be no Caucasian gender differences in fracture rates, although there are clear differences in prevalence rates when calculating T score from a male vs. female reference population database, as would be expected from the basic analysis of the T-score equation. Small differences in the SD of the reference population database profoundly affect the subsequent T-score calculation.[19,20] It is for this reason that whenever T scores are calculated from two different, yet seemingly young and healthy, reference population databases, the T score calculated in the same patient will invariably differ. As mentioned, the only consistent young-normal reference population database between BMD machines is the NHANES III database for the central DXA hip, which is why the T score is the same among all three central DXA manufacturers in the same patient measuring the hip.[21]

The percentage of men with T scores <−2.5 at the femoral neck when the T score is calculated from a male database is 6%; from the female database it is 4%. As far as the hip prevalence is concerned, few differences exist between the two different databases when it comes to prevalence comparing T scores in men calculated from a male or female reference population database. Thus, in consideration of the hip alone, the small differences in prevalence between the two genders using NHANES III databases will not miss many men at risk. On the other hand, when the prevalence of osteoporosis by WHO criteria is determined in men from a male vs. female database and the prevalence is determined by adding the spine, wrist, and hip measurements, the prevalence in men is 19% when the T score is calculated from a male database and 6% when calculated from a female database.[22,23] Thus, as far as prevalence (diagnosis) is concerned, men are *Underdiagnosed* if the clinician is examining multiple skeletal sites, when their SD (T) scores are calculated from a female database. Therefore, the number of men determined to be at risk for fracture would be underestimated by combining all three central DXA measured skeletal sites, if a female reference population database were used. It is for this reason that the recent International Society for Clinical Densitometry (ISCD) Position Development Conference recommended that a gender-specific reference database be used to calculate T scores.[24] It will take head-to-head trials looking at volumetric BMD (which takes into account bone size) and a real BMD assessed by DXA (which does not take into account the size of the bone with fracture outcomes) to really know whether there are differences in fracture risk between the genders as a function of bone size.[25,26]

In contrast to equal prevalence of vertebral fractures between men and women, a recent longitudinal study of incident vertebral fractures in Caucasian men vs. Caucasian women suggests that incident fractures are twice as frequent in women as in men.[27–29] The reasons for incident differences in vertebral fractures are unknown, because when one examines the known risk factors for age-related incident vertebral fractures, only three have an influence: age, BMD, and prevalent vertebral fracture.

In summary, with regard to the gender issues, prevalence is highly dependent on gender-specific databases. Hip fracture risk may be the same (5–10 years) between Caucasian men and women with either absolute BMD of the hip or T scores derived from the female Caucasian reference database. Vertebral fracture incidence rates seem to differ between the two genders, although in the only head-to-head between gender study, the absolute BMD predicted the same vertebral fracture incidence in men and women.[30]

Ethnic Differences

What about ethnic differences? The only head-to-head ethnic comparison in which both T and Z scores (number of SDs a patient's BMD is above or below the age-matched population) were calculated from both gender- and ethnic-specific consistent databases for prevalence comparisons is the NHANES III reference database. Here, ethnic-specific databases were calculated from Caucasian, Hispanic, and African-American male and female populations between the ages of 20 and 80 years. There were no Asians in the NHANES III database. In this robust study, there are clear prevalence differences if a different ethnic group's T or Z scores are calculated from a nonethnic-specific database. Yet there are no fracture data correlated to these T or Z scores from the NHANES III database. Hence, we have no data as to whether there are differences in fracture rates as a function of the ethnicity-derived T scores from this valuable dataset.

The only multiethnic head-to-head prevalence and fracture data again come from NORA, in which all SD scores were calculated from the Caucasian-female reference population database. The RR/SD for global fractures were similar between the U.S. multiethnic groups of Caucasian, American-Hispanic, and Native-American, and lower in the American-Asian and African-American population.[31] On the other hand, the fracture rates across all these ethnicities at T scores <−2.5 was similar (Fig. 3-5).[31] In the WHO-defined osteopenic category in NORA

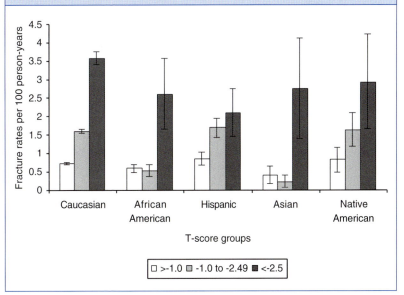

Figure 3-5. Fracture rates by ethnicity and T-score group. (Data from Barrett-Conner E, Siris E, Wehren L, et al. Low bone mass and fracture risk in women of different ethnic groups: results from the National Osteoporosis Risk Assessment (NORA). J Bone Miner Res, 2004 [submitted].)

across ethnicities, the American-Asians were unexpectedly low in fracture events. The reason Asians have lower fracture rates is unclear. There are severeal possible explanations, including lower bone turnover and shorter hip-axis length. To the extent, however, that all the risk calculations in NORA were done from a Caucasian female reference population database and that fracture rates were not too dissimilar across ethnicities, at least for the U.S. multiethnic female postmenopausal population, it might be acceptable to calculate risk from a Caucasian female database, regardless of the American ethnicity. Native Chinese have a lower hip fracture risk (yet similar vertebral fracture risk) despite having a much lower absolute BMD, even after adjusting for body mass index (BMI).[32] It is possible that in the United States our lifestyle, nutrition, or some element of the gene-pool mix contribute to the similar fracture rates observed in all ethic groups. What does this mean, and what does the ISCD endorse? Until we have ethnic-specific databases in all BMD manufacturers and these prevalence data are linked to risk assessment, the ISCD suggests the use of nonethnic-adjusted databases for T-score calculation[33–35] available, in a given BMD device. Yet, if a physician has a BMD device without any ethnic-specific database and, for example, has a patient whose ethnicity is not available in a specific BMD device, the physician.

Key Points: Osteoporosis Fractures

- ↜ Low BMD is a powerful predictor of fracture risk in postmenopausal women and elderly men.
- ↜ The three most powerful risk factors are low BMD, increasing age, and prevalent vertebral fracture. In addition, falling is an important risk factor for hip fracture.
- ↜ Male databases should be used for T-score calculation in men to determine both prevalence and risk prediction.
- ↜ Use ethnic-specific databases, if available, for the determination of prevalence and risk among ethnicities. If an ethnic-specific database is not available in any given BMD measuring device, then use a Caucasian database for risk prediction.

References

1. WHO Study Group: Assessment of Fracture Risk and its Application to Screening for Postmenopausal Osteoporosis. World Health Organization, Geneva, Switzerland, 1994.
2. Miller PD, Njeh CF, Jankowski LG, et al: What are the standards by which bone mass measurements at peripheral skeletal sites should be used in the diagnosis of osteoporosis? J Clin Densitom 5(Suppl):S39–S46, 2002.

3. McMahon K, Kalnins S, Freund J, et al: Discordance in lumbar spine T scores and non-standardization of standard deviations. J Clin Densitom 6:1, 2002.

4. Faulkner KG, Roberts L, McClung M: Discrepancies in normative data between Lunar and Hologic DXA systems. Osteoporosis Inter 6:432–436, 1996.

5. Hui SL, Slemenda CW, Johnston CC Jr: Age and bone mass as predictors of fracture in a prospective study. J Clin Invest 81:1804–1809, 1988.

6. Marshall D, Johnell O, Wedel H: Meta-analysis of how well measurements of bone mineral density predict the occurrence of osteoporotic fractures. BMJ 312:1254–1259, 1996.

7. Cummings S, Black D, Nevitt M, et al: Bone density at various sites for prediction of hip fractures. The study of osteoporotic fractures research group. Lancet 341:72–75, 1993.

8. Bauer D, Gluer C, Cauley JA, et al: Broadband ultrasound attenuation predicts fractures strongly and independently of densitometry in older women. Arch Intern Med 157:629–634, 1997.

9. Siris ES, Miller PD, Barrett-Conner E, et al: Identification and fracture outcomes of undiagnosed low bone mineral density in post-menopausal women: results from the National Osteoporosis Risk Assessment (NORA). JAMA 286:2815–2822, 2000.

10. Miller PD, Siris ES, Barrett-Conner E, et al: Prediction of fracture risk in post-menopausal Caucasian women with peripheral bone densitometry: Evidence from the National Osteoporosis Risk Assessment (NORA). J Bone Miner Res 17: 2222–2230, 2002.

11. Ross PD, Davis JW, Epstein RS, et al: Pre-existing fracture and bone mass predict vertebral fracture incidence in women. Ann Intern Med 114:919–923, 1998.

12. Tinetti ME: Preventing falls in elderly persons. N Engl J Med 348:42–49, 2003.

13. Ruff CB, Hayes WC. Sex differences in age-related modeling of the femur and tibia. J Orthop Res 6:886–896, 1988.

14. Cummings SR, Nevitt MC, Browner WS, et al: Risk factors for hip fracture in white women. N Engl J Med 332:76, 1995.

15. Kanis JA, Johnell O, Oden A, et al: Interventional thresholds for osteoporosis. Bone 31:26–31, 2002.

16. Kanis JA: Risk factors for hip fracture. Osteoporos Int 11:120, 2000.

17. De Laet CEDH, Van Hout BA, Burger H, et al: Hip fracture prediction in elderly men and women: validation in the Rotterdam study. J Bone Miner Res 13:1587–1593, 1998.

18. Kanis JA, Johnell O, Oden A, et al: Ten year probabilities of osteoporotic fractures according to BMD and diagnostic thresholds. J Bone Miner Res 16:S1, 2001.

19. Ahmed AIH, Blake GM, Rymer JM, et al: Screening for osteopoenia and osteoporosis: do the accepted normal ranges lead to overdiagnosis? Osteoporos Int 7:432–438, 1997.

20. Faulkner KG, VonStetten E, Miler PD: Discordance in patient classification using T scores. J Clin Densitom 2:343–350, 1990.

21. Looker AC, Wahner HW, Dunn WL, et al: Proximal femur bone mineral levels of US adults. Osteoporos Int 5:389–409, 1995.

22. Melton LJ III, Atkinson EJ, O'Conner MK, et al: Bone densitometry and fracture risk in men. J Bone Miner Res 13:1915–1923, 1998.

23. Vallarta-Ast N, Krueger D, Binkley N: Densitometric diagnosis of osteoporosis in men. J Clin Densitom 5:383–389, 2003.

24. Binkley NC, Schmeer P, Wasnich RD, et al: What are the criteria by which a densitometric diagnosis of osteoporosis can be made in males and non-caucasians? J Clin Densitom 5:S19–S28, 2002.

25. Orwoll E: Assessing bone density in men. J Bone Miner Res 15:1867–1870, 2000.

26. Seeman E: An exercise in geometry. J Bone Miner Res 17:373–380, 2002.

27. McCloskey EV, Spector TD, Eyers KS: The assessment of vertebral deformity: a method for use in population studies and clinical trials. Osteoporosis Int 3:138–147, 1993.
28. O'Neill TW, Felsenberg D, Varlow J, et al: The prevalence of vertebral deformity in European women and men: The European Vertebral Osteoporosis Study (EVOS). J Bone Miner Res 11:1010–1017, 1996.
29. Roy DK, O'Neill TW, Finn JD, et al: Determinants of incident vertebral fracture in men and women: results from the European Prospective Osteoporosis Study (EPOS). J Bone Miner Res 16:720–724, 2002.
30. Huang C, Ross PD, Wasnich RD: Short-term and long-term fracture prediction by bone mass measurements: a prospective study. J Bone Miner Res 13:107–113, 1998.
31. Barrett-Conner E , Siris E, Wehren L, et al: Low bone mass and fracture risk in women of different ethnic groups: results from the National Osteoporosis Risk Assessment (NORA). J Bone Miner Res, 2004 (submitted).
32. Cummings SR, Cauley JA, Palmero L, et al: Racial differences in hip axis lengths might explain racial differences in rates of hip fracture. Study of Osteoporotic Fractures Research Group. Osteoporos Int 4(4):226–229, 1994.
33. Miller PD, Bilezikian JP: Bone densitometry in asymptomatic primary hyperparathyroidism. J Bone Miner Res 17(Suppl. 2): N98–N102, 2002.
34. Miller PD: Controversial issues in bone densitometry. In Bilezikian JP, Raisz L, Rodan G. (eds.): Principles of Bone Biology ed. New York, Academic Press, 2002, pp. 1587–1597.
35. Leib ES, Lewiecki EM, Binkley N, et al: Official positions of the International Society for Clinical Densitometry. J Clin Densit 7(1):1–5, 2004.

Diagnosis of Osteoporosis

chapter
4

Paul D. Miller, M.D.

The clinical application of bone densitometry has been one of the advances in the field of osteoporosis that has led to the increased patient awareness of this increasingly prevalent disease.[1,2] Bone densitometry has made it possible for clinicians to diagnose osteoporosis before the first fracture has occurred; predict risk for fracture in postmenopausal women, men, and patients receiving glucocorticoids; and to be used as a surrogate marker to follow the efficacy of therapies and to examine those patients who might be osteoporosis-specific therapeutic nonresponders.[3–7]

Hence, there are three reasons clinicians do BMD measurements:

1. Diagnosis using the World Health Organization (WHO) criteria for osteoporosis

2. Fracture risk prediction

3. Monitoring the natural progression of diseases that affect BMD or monitoring the therapeutic response to osteoporosis-specific treatments.

Diagnosis by WHO Criteria

In 1994, the WHO selected a BMD cut-point for defining the prevalence of osteoporosis in the Caucasian postmenopausal female population.[8] The main intent of the WHO committee was to assess the prevalence of low bone mass in the population and relate this bone mass to the anticipated lifetime fracture risk to advise health policymakers of what the anticipated medical and economic burden of osteoporotic fractures might become in this population. The use of standard deviation (SD) scores (T score) rather than absolute BMD in g/cm^2 was decided on because of the known different absolute BMD calibrations that existed between the then-existing BMD measuring devices. A SD score mitigates some of the variance between absolute BMD between manufacturer devices.

The WHO cutoff point of T −2.5 or lower used for the diagnosis of osteoporosis was based on a close association between prevalence at this cutoff point and lifetime fracture risk of hip fractures or all fractures (hip, vertebrae, forearm, humerus, and pelvis). At the femoral neck as assessed by the young-normal reference population database, 16% of postmenopausal women 50 years of age and older are at or <−2.5 SD, and the lifetime fracture risk from age 50 years in postmenopausal Caucasian women is 16%. In addition, the percentage (prevalence) of this population at or <−2.5 SD measuring the hip, spine, and wrist is ~ 30%, which approximates the lifetime fracture risk of all previously described "all" or global fractures from the age of 50. However, the relationship between low BMD and increased fracture risk is a gradient and not a threshold. With that knowledge in mind, the WHO created a separate classification, osteopenia, to recognize this gradient of risk and to help clinicians assess additional risk factors that may lead to increased fracture risk above and beyond that risk based on the level of BMD alone. In that regard, in the recently published National Osteoporosis and Risk Assessment (NORA) dataset, although the 1-year fracture rates and relative risk for fracture/SD reduction in BMD was greatest at T scores −2.5 SD or less, the largest number of fractures in NORA, partially related to the larger sample size of the population with T scores between −1.0 and −2.5 SD, was seen in this osteopenic category (Fig. 4-1).[9,10]

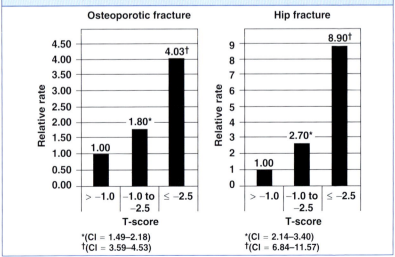

Figure 4-1. Risk for fracture in the National Osteoporosis Risk Assessment in postmenopausal women as a function of the T score. (Data from Siris ES, Miller PD, Barrett-Conner E, et al. Identification and fracture outcomes of undiagnosed low bone mineral density in post-menopausal women: results from the National Osteoporosis Risk Assessment (NORA). JAMA 286:2815–2822, 2001.)

Low BMD in the postmenopausal population assessed by any BMD device and by any database is predictive of an increased fracture risk if the value is low; this relationship is also seen in the multiethnic U.S. population (Fig. 4-2).[11] Yet, for various reasons the values (T scores) obtained by peripheral devices may not always be as low as T scores determined from central DXA devices (Fig. 4-3).[12] The major reason behind this underdetection of osteopenia or osteoporosis is inconsistent young-normal reference population databases from which the T scores are calculated: peripheral devices seem to underestimate the prevalence, so fewer people may be detected as having low BMD by peripheral devices that would have been low by central DXA devices (Fig. 4-3).[12]

The prevalence of WHO osteoporosis (T <−2.5) in the NORA dataset of postmenopausal women 50 years of age and older averaged 7% using all four peripheral devices combined, half of the prevalence determined from the WHO dataset in postmenopausal women measuring only the femoral neck (16%) (Fig. 4-4).[10,13] Thus, although a low peripheral BMD does predict an increase in fracture risk, any T-score

Figure 4-2. Fracture rates across ethnicities according to T-score classsification 1-year follow-up data from the National Osteoporosis Risk Assessment (NORA). (Data from Barrett-Conner E, Siris E, Wehren L, et al. Low bone mass and fracture risk in women of different ethnic groups: results from the National Osteoporosis Risk Assessment (NORA). J Bone Miner Res, 2004 [submitted].)

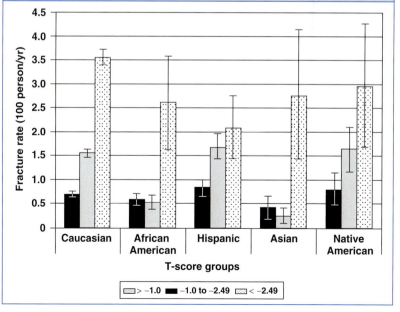

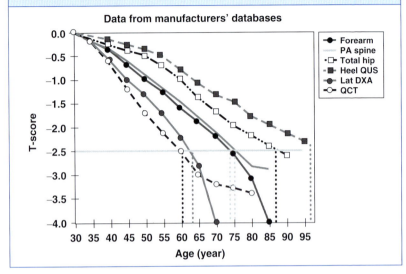

Figure 4-3. T scores by different bone mass measurement devices according to age and the WHO criteria. (Data from Faulkner KG, VonStetten E, Miller PD. Discordance in patient classification using T scores. J Clin Densitom 2:343–350, 1999.)

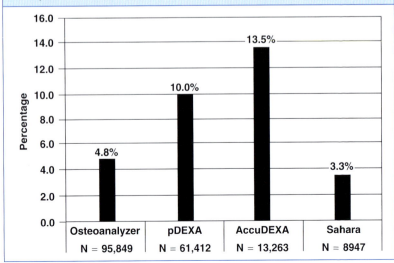

Figure 4-4. Lower prevalence of WHO-defined osteoporosis by peripheral devices in NORA in postmenopausal women. (Data from Miller PD, Siris ES, Barrett-Conner E, et al. Prediction of fracture risk in postmenopausal Caucasian women with peripheral bone densitometry: evidence from the National Osteoporosis Risk Assessment (NORA). J Bone Miner Res 17:2222–2230, 2002.)

number can only be predictive if the value is found to be low. Thus, clinicians interpreting peripheral BMD computer printout reports should guide recommendations to follow up a normal peripheral BMD with a central BMD measurement if the patient has additional risk factors that would lead the clinician to believe that there could be a low central DXA BMD.[14] These discrepancies between T-score calculations among various BMD devices are well recognized and still exist at the spine and wrist between different central DXA manufacture's skeletal sites using central DXA technologies as well.[15]

T-score discrepancies had previously existed at the hip due to use of the three central DXA manufacturer-specific reference databases, until it was shown that calculating the T scores at the hip from the only consistent reference population databases, NHANES III, eliminated the hip T-score discrepancy.[16] In fact, before NHANES III was installed as the default device in all three central DXA manufacturers, there was a 1.0 SD difference between Hologic vs Lunar–GE T scores at the hip.[16] When clinical trial outcomes were reassessed later with the NHANES III dataset, whereas the original randomization had been accomplished with the manufacturer-specific reference population database, many patients who had previously been assumed to have WHO osteoporosis now had WHO osteopenia, and pharmacologic outcomes became altered as a function of changing the patients but not the dataset.[17]

This issue of divergent T scores yielding inconsistent WHO classification becomes even more compounded among peripheral manufacturers. Different peripheral devices yield dissimilar prevalences of WHO-defined osteoporosis or osteopenia,[18–29] not so much as a function of the heterogeneity of the type of bone structures peripheral devices measure as the fact that their individual T scores are all calculated from each manufacturer-specific reference population database. It is for this reason that the peripheral bone-measuring technologies cannot be used for the diagnosis of osteoporosis or osteopenia.[30] The development of a standardized young-normal reference population database would do much to mitigate T-score discrepancies between central and peripheral devices and unify the WHO diagnosis between central and peripheral devices.[31–33] Support for the validity of this concept has been the development of data showing that the use of a consistent young-normal database mitigated the T-score discrepancies that existed between different BMD measuring devices: both central and peripheral (heel ultrasound, heel DXA, hip DXA), when the T score is calculated from a consistent database.[20]

In the meantime, when a clinician is faced with different T scores obtained on different machines in the same patient, the fundamental question is: Doctor, do I have or do I not have osteoporosis? Until these T-score discrepancies can be resolved, the clinician's best response is to base opinion on evidence that the probability of being <−2.5 SD at the hip when the heel ultrasound measurement is > −1.0 is small (<10%), and the probability of a hip T score being <−1.0 if a heel T score is 0 is also small. On the other hand, if the heel ultra-sound is <−1.0 SD, the likelihood that a hip is <−2.5 is high (70%). In the absence of central DXA access, clinical decisions about risk assessment and interventions might be considered, especially in patients 50 years of age and older if a peripheral T score is <−1.0 SD. Alternately, if the physician has uncertainty about a particular T score value and needs confirmation, central DXA should be performed, if available. Even though in the United States there are approximately 15,000 central DXA devices available, many urban elderly people or rural people of all age ranges have limited access to these "gold-stan-dard" devices.

The other means of trying to equate different T scores from differ-ent BMD devices is a project spearheaded by the National Osteoporosis Foundation (NOF) and the International Society for Clinical Densitometry (ISCD). This project is called "The T-score Equivalence."[34] The fundamental concept behind this project is to select a device-specific T-score cutoff that predicts the same 5-year hip fracture risk as that risk predicted from the femoral neck T score at −2.5 as determined by the NHANES III reference population data-base.[35] NHANES III is the only consistent database in existence. It exists only for the hip DXA measurements and is now the default database in all central DXA manufacturers. Most of the data for T-score equivalence is derived from the SOF, one of the largest prospective epidemiologic fracture studies in postmenopausal women in the United States.[5] In SOF, for example at the age of 70 years, the 5-year hip fracture risk as determined by a T score of −2.5 SD at the femoral neck is 5%. Using, for example, the heel ultra-sound device manufactured by Hologic, a manufacturer-specific database-derived T score at the same age of 70 years predicts the equal 5-year hip fracture risk of 5% at a T score of −2.0. Hence, if a physician had only the Sahara heel ultrasound available and the patient (age-specific) had a T score as determined on the Sahara that predicts the equal hip fracture risk as if the patient had a hip DXA performed at a T score of −2.5, this specific heel T score would become the value for the diagnosis of osteoporosis (i.e., for the 70-year-old example, −2.0 by ultrasound and −2.5 by femoral neck). In this way, the physician with a specific peripheral device could use a different T-score cutoff point for the diagnosis of osteoporosis, because it predicted an equal risk as a −2.5 by the femoral neck as assessed by the NHANES III database. This short-term solution to the T-score discrepancy problem has the support of both the scientific societies and the Food and Drug Administration (FDA) regulatory-device division.

Despite some limitations, the T-score equivalency project offers the best short-term answer to the clinical application of the T-score discrepancy problem.

Abandonment of the T score has been suggested for all BMD devices and skeletal sites with the exception of the hip T score, with the use of all other skeletal sites and BMD/ultrasound technologies only for fracture risk assessment.[36] If we abandon the T score, what will we replace it with? Absolute BMD in g/cm^2 values also differs between BMD devices of different manufacturers, even when measuring the same skeletal site and the "same" region of interest. This is true both for the peripheral devices previously mentioned and for central DXA devices. For example, the average BMD of the axial skeleton (L2–L4) in a healthy 20-year-old Caucasian woman is 1.25 g/cm^2 by Lunar-GE and 1.00 g/cm^2 for the same patient. These different BMD values are related to the different calibrations of the two manufacturers. Because there are so many devices that yield inconsistent absolute BMD values, there is no standardized BMD between all devices related either to prevalence or fracture risk. A standardized BMD does exist for the three central DXA devices for the spine and hip.[37,38] This was developed by performing duplicate BMD measurements in 100 postmenopausal women, and, through use of a linear regression, deriving a mathematical equation that reduces much of the absolute BMD between the three central DXA manufacturers. In the newer central DXA computer printout reports, the standard BMD (sBMD) should automatically be calculated at the bottom of the page for the clinician to compare absolute BMD between manufacturers. Although this standardized BMD helps in the serial monitoring of patients that move from one manufacturer to another, there are no data relating sBMD to fracture risk prediction. Furthermore, no sBMD exists for the wrist by central DXA or any of the multiple peripheral devices. Once the universal, standardized database is completed for both the young-normal reference population database and the older population with and without spine and hip fractures on all FDA-approved devices, a common standardized BMD value can also be calculated between devices, with this single standardized BMD number derived from all central and peripheral devices now also linked to fracture risk prediction.

Key Points: Diagnosis of Osteoporosis

☞ Low bone density is a highly predictive factor for future fracture risk in the early and late postmenopausal population.

☞ Both central DXA and peripheral bone density measuring technologies can equally predict the risk for fragility (hip and nonhip) fractures in postmenopausal women.

☞ T-score discrepancies (largely because of nonstandardization of reference population databases) exist between all peripheral devices, as well as central DXA spine and hip measurements. These T-score discrepancies lead to a different WHO classification between peripheral devices and central forearm and spine devices. T-score discrepancies lead to significant diagnostic issues for patient classification (i.e., osteoporosis or osteopenia) and decisions concerning when to start therapy with osteoporosis-specific pharmacologic therapeutics.

☞ Yet, if a T score is <1.0 SD in a peripheral device measurement, the risk for both hip fracture and all (global) fractures is increased.

References

1. Miller PD, Bonnick SL: Clinical application of bone densitometry. In Favus M (ed): Primer on the Metabolic Bone Diseases and Disorders of Mineral Metabolism, 4th ed. Philadelphia, Lippincott Williams & Wilkins, 1999, pp 152–159.
2. Miller PD, Bonnick SL, Rosen CJ: Clinical utility of bone mass measurements in adults: consensus of an international panel. Semin Arthritis Rheum 25:361–372, 1996.
3. Ross PD, Davis JW, Epstein RS, et al: Pre-existing fracture and bone mass predict vertebral fracture incidence in women. Ann Intern Med 114:919–923, 1998.
4. Ross PD, Genant HK, Davis JW, et al: Predicting vertebral fracture incidence from prevalent fractures and bone density among non-black osteoporotic women. Osteoporos Int 3:120–126, 1993.
5. Cummings S, Black D, Nevitt M, et al: Bone density at various sites for prediction of hip fractures. The study of osteoporotic fractures research group. Lancet 341:72–75, 1993.
6. Miller PD, McClung M: Prediction of fracture risk I: Bone density. Am J Med Sci 312:257–259, 1996.
7. Miller PD, Zapalowski C, Kulak CAM, et al: Bone densitometry: the best way to detect osteoporosis and to monitor therapy. J Clin Endocrinol Metab 84:1867–1871, 1999.
8. WHO Study Group: Assessment of fracture risk and its application to screening for postmenopausal osteoporosis. World Health Organization, Geneva, Switzerland, 1994.
9. Siris ES, Miller PD, Barrett-Conner E, et al: Identification and fracture outcomes of undiagnosed low bone mineral density in post-menopausal women: results from the National Osteoporosis Risk Assessment (NORA). JAMA 286:2815–2822, 2001.
10. Miller PD, Siris ES, Barrett-Conner E, et al: Prediction of fracture risk in postmenopausal Caucasian women with peripheral bone densitometry: evidence from the National Osteoporosis Risk Assessment (NORA). J Bone Miner Res 17:2222–2230, 2002.

11. Barrett-Conner E , Siris E, Wehren L, et al: Low bone mass and fracture risk in women of different ethnic groups: Results from the National Osteoporosis Risk Assessment (NORA). J Bone Miner Res, 2004 (submitted).

12. Faulkner KG, VonStetten E, Miller PD: Discordance in patient classification using T scores. J Clin Densitom 2:343–350, 1990.

13. Melton LJ III. How many women have osteoporosis now? J Bone Miner Res 10:175–177, 1995.

14. Miller PD, Bonnick SL, Johnston CC Jr, et al: The challenges of peripheral densitometry: which patients need additional central density skeletal measurements? J Clin Densitom 1:211–217, 1998.

15. McMahon K, Kalnins S, Freund J, et al: Discordance in lumbar spine T scores and non-standardization of standard deviations. J Clin Densitom 6:1–6, 2003.

16. Faulkner KG, Roberts L, McClung M: Discrepancies in normative data between Lunar and Hologic DXA systems. Osteoporos Int 6:432–436, 1996.

17. Miller PD: Greater risk, greater benefit: true or false (editorial). J Clin Endocrinol Metab 88:538–541, 2003.

18. Blake GM, Fogelman I: Peripheral or central densitometry: does it matter which technique we use. J Clin Densitom 4:83–96, 2001.

19. Drake WM, McClung M, Njeh CF, et al: Multisite bone ultrasound measurement on North American female reference population. J Clin Densitom 4:239–248, 2001.

20. Greenspan SL, Cheng S, Miller PD, Orwoll E (for the QUS-2 PMA Trials Group): Clinical performance of a highly portable, scanning calcaneal ultrasonometer. Osteoporos Int 12:391–398, 2001.

21. Greenspan SL Bouxsein ML, Melton ME, et al: Precision and discriminatory ability of calcaneal bone assessment technologies. J Bone Miner Res 12:1301–1313, 1997.

22. Lippuner K, Fuchs G, Ruetsche AG, et al: How well do radiographic absorptiometry and quantitative ultrasound predict osteoporosis at spine or hip? J Clin Densitom 3:241–249, 2000.

23. Lu Y, Genant HK, Shepherd J, et al: Classification of osteoporosis based on bone mineral densities. J Bone Miner Res 16:901–910, 2001.

24. Mulder JE, Michaeli D, Flaster ER, et al: Comparison of bone mineral density of the phalanges, lumbar spine, hip and forearm for assessment of osteoporosis in postmenopausal women. J Clin Densitom 4:373–381, 2000.

25. Nelson DA, Molloy R , Kleerekoper M: Prevalence of osteoporosis in women referred for bone density testing. J Clin Densitom 1:5–11, 1998.

26. Shepherd J, Cheng XO, Lu Y, et al: Universal standardization of forearm bone densitometry. J Bone Miner Res 17:734–745, 2002.

27. Sweeny AT, Malabanan AO, Blake MA, et al: Bone mineral density assessment: comparison of dual-energy x-ray absorptiometry measurements at the calcaneus, spine and hip. J Clin Densitom 5:57–62, 2002.

28. Arlot ME, Sornay-Rendu E, Garnero P, et al: Apparent pre- and postmenopausal bone loss evaluated by DXA at different skeletal sites in women: the OFLEY cohort. J Bone Miner Res 12:683–690, 1997.

29. Cummings SR, Palmero L, Black DM: Using forearm BMD to find osteoporosis at the hip. J Bone Miner Res 16:S340, 2001.

30. Miller PD, Njeh CF, Jankowski LG, et al: What are the standards by which bone mass measurements at peripheral skeletal sites should be used in the diagnosis of osteoporosis ? J Clin Densitom 5(Suppl): S39–S46, 2002.

31. Miller PD: Controversies in bone mineral density diagnostic classifications. Calcif Tissue Int 66:317–319, 2000.

32. Miller PD: Controversial issues in bone densitometry. In Bilezikian JP, Raisz L, Rodan G (eds): Principles of Bone Biology, 2nd ed. New York, Academic Press, 2002, pp 1587–1597.
33. Simmons A, Simpson DE, O'Doherty MJ, et al: The effects of standardization and reference values on patient classification for spine and femur dual-energy x-ray absorptiometry. Osteoporos Int 7:200–206, 1997.
34. Black D, Johnston CC Jr, Palmero L, et al: A proposal to establish comparable diagnostic categories for bone densitometry based on hip fracture risk among Caucasian women over age 65 years. J Bone Miner Res 16:S342, 2001.
35. Looker AC, Wahner HW, Dunn WL, et al: Proximal femur bone mineral levels of US adults. Osteoporos Int 5:389–409, 1995.
36. Kanis JA, Gluer CC: An update on the diagnosis and assessment of osteoporosis with densitometry. Osteoporos Int 11:192–202, 2000.
37. Hanson J: Standardization of proximal femur bone mineral density (BMD) measurements by DXA. Committee for standards in DXA. J Bone Miner Res 12:1316–1317, 1997.
38. Steiger P: Standardization of spine BMD measurements. J Bone Miner Res 10:1602–1603, 1995.

Evaluation of the Patient with Low Bone Mass or Fragility Fracture

chapter

5

Michael T. McDermott, M.D.

Assessing the Cause of Low Bone Mass

Once a person is diagnosed with low bone mass or has sustained a fragility fracture, further evaluation is indicated to determine whether there is an underlying condition or disease that contributes to or is responsible for the bone disease. Although peak bone mass and the rate of postmenopausal and age-related bone loss certainly have important genetic (primary) determinants, conditions causing secondary bone loss have been reported in up to 30% of women[1,2] and 64% of men[3] with osteoporosis. Table 5-1 lists the conditions most commonly identified.[1–5] Some of these cause typical osteoporosis, whereas others cause bone disease that is histologically distinct from true osteoporosis but that nevertheless causes diminished bone strength, predisposing to skeletal fractures. These conditions are important to identify, because they may signify the presence of a serious underlying systemic disease and because they may respond to specific therapy aside from the usual measures used to treat osteoporosis.

The initial evaluation should begin with a complete history and physical examination, followed by several laboratory tests that are considered to be cost-effective[2] (Table 5-2). When these tests are normal in a patient with otherwise typical osteoporosis, no further evaluation is usually necessary. More extensive testing should be considered in men, in premenopausal women, and in patients who have abnormalities on the initial assessment. Patients with elevated serum calcium levels should have a serum intact parathyroid hormone (PTH) measurement. An elevated or high normal serum PTH value associated with hypercalcemia indicates the presence of primary hyperparathyroidism (Fig. 5-1). A low or undetectable PTH value associated with hypercalcemia merits further

Table 5-1. Risk Factors for Low Bone Mass

Nutritional/lifestyle factors
- Low calcium intake
- Low vitamin D intake
- Cigarette smoking
- Alcohol excess
- Caffeine excess
- Sedentary lifestyle
- Immobilization

Endocrine disorders
- Hyperparathyroidism
- Hyperthyroidism
- Hypogonadism
- Hyperprolactinemia
- Cushing's syndrome

Gastrointestinal disorders
- Celiac disease
- Inflammatory bowel disease
- Hepatobiliary disease
- Malabsorption syndromes
- Hemochromatosis

Renal diseases
- Chronic renal failure
- Idiopathic hypercalciuria
- Renal tubular acidosis

Bone marrow disorders
- Multiple myeloma
- Lymphoma/leukemia
- Systemic mastocytosis

Connective tissue disorders
- Rheumatoid arthritis
- Systemic lupus erythematosus
- Osteogenesis imperfecta
- Marfan's syndrome

Medications
- Glucocorticoids
- Thyroxine excess
- Anticonvulsants
- Heparin
- Cyclosporin

Table 5-2. Evaluation of the Patient Who Has Low Bone Mass or a Fragility Fracture

History and physical examination
Routine laboratory testing
- CBC, erythrocyte sedimentation rate
- Serum calcium, phosphorus, creatinine, alkaline phosphatase
- Serum testosterone (men)
- 24-hour urine calcium, creatinine

Selected laboratory testing
- Serum PTH
- Serum 25 hydroxyvitamin D
- Serum TSH
- Serum prolactin
- Serum estradiol, LH, FSH
- 24-hour urine cortisol
- Serum/urine protein electrophoresis
- Serum transglutaminase antibodies
- Small bowel biopsy
- Bone or bone marrow biopsy

Figure 5-1. **Primary hyperparathyroidism** is one condition that is associated with secondary bone loss. In this disorder, excess parathyroid hormone (PTH) is secreted by a solitary parathyroid adenoma (85% of cases) or by four-gland parathyroid hyperplasia (15% of cases). Excess PTH stimulates bone resorption, renal calcium retention, and intestinal calcium absorption (through increased renal 1,25 [OH]2 vitamin D production), causing an increase in the serum calcium concentration. The key to making this diagnosis is the finding of an elevated serum calcium level in association with a high or high-normal serum PTH level. The definitive treatment for moderate and severe cases is parathyroidectomy.

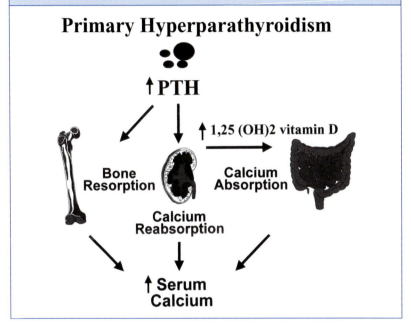

Primary Hyperparathyroidism

↑PTH

↑ 1,25 (OH)2 vitamin D

Bone Resorption

Calcium Absorption

Calcium Reabsorption

↑ Serum Calcium

evaluation with a chest x-ray, serum protein electrophoresis, 25 hydroxyvitamin D measurement, and, in some cases, a parathyroid hormone–related protein (PTHrp) level to investigate the possibility of underlying malignancy, granulomatous disease, and vitamin D toxicity. Elevated urinary calcium excretion (>300 mg/day) should prompt a similar evaluation, because hypercalciuria alone may occur in milder forms of these same conditions; the absence of other abnormal findings indicates a probable diagnosis of idiopathic hypercalciuria in these patients.

Low serum calcium levels, particularly in association with low serum phosphorus and elevated alkaline phosphatase levels, suggest the presence of overt vitamin D deficiency and resultant osteomalacia. Low urinary calcium excretion (<100 mg/day) with normal serum calcium levels may be an early indicator of a more subtle vitamin D deficiency caused by intestinal malabsorption or inadequate dietary vitamin D and/or calcium intake. Secondary hyperparathyroidism (low or low-normal serum calcium levels associated with elevated serum PTH values) is often present in these circumstances and contributes significantly to the ongoing bone loss (Fig. 5-2). Patients with these findings should have their daily calcium consumption, vitamin D intake, and sunlight exposure carefully assessed. Blood testing for serum 25 hydroxyvitamin D levels and tissue transglutaminase antibodies (for celiac disease) should follow. Depending on the results, small bowel biopsies or radiographic studies for seronegative celiac disease and other intestinal disorders should also be considered.

Figure 5-2. Secondary hyperparathyroidism is another cause of secondary bone loss. This condition, which can have many causes, commonly occurs when there is deficient dietary calcium and/or vitamin D intake or intestinal malabsorption, causing a reduction in the serum calcium concentration. Parathyroid hyperplasia with increased parathyroid hormone (PTH) secretion occurs as a compensatory mechanism to maintain the serum calcium level in the normal range. The key to this diagnosis is the finding of a low or low-normal serum calcium level associated with an elevated serum PTH level. Treatment must be aimed at correction of the calcium and vitamin D deficiencies.

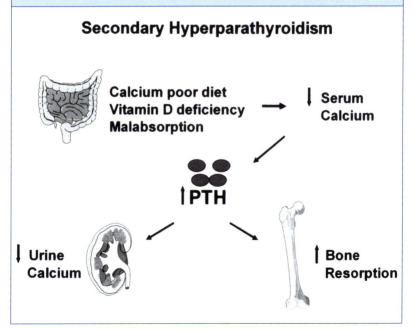

Secondary Hyperparathyroidism

Calcium poor diet
Vitamin D deficiency
Malabsorption
→ ↓ Serum Calcium

↑PTH

↓ Urine Calcium

↑ Bone Resorption

Patients who have clinical features suggesting thyroid dysfunction should have their serum TSH measured. Individuals with Cushingoid features and those with unusually low bone mass should also have a 24-hour urinary cortisol measurement. Premenopausal women with osteoporosis should have additional testing of serum prolactin, estradiol (E2), and follicle-stimulating hormone (FSH) to evaluate their gonadal axis. An elevated serum FSH and low E2 suggest premature menopause. An elevated serum prolactin and/or a low serum E2 and FSH suggest pituitary disease and should be followed by MRI testing. Men with osteoporosis and low serum testosterone levels should have further measurement of serum prolactin and luteinizing hormone (LH). An elevated serum LH usually indicates primary gonadal failure, whereas an elevated prolactin or low LH suggests pituitary disease, which should be further assessed with an MRI and serum iron studies (for hemochromatosis).

Bone biopsy and bone marrow biopsy infrequently yield a diagnosis that is not already apparent after the preceding tests are completed. However, rare disorders, such as systemic mastocytosis, may only be discovered by histologic examination of the bone marrow. This procedure may therefore be indicated when the etiology of the bone disorder has otherwise remained elusive. Osteogenesis imperfecta, a congenital disorder caused by a defect in procollagen synthesis, can be diagnosed definitively only by genetic testing. The diagnosis is suspected clinically by the finding of blue-tinged sclerae and a history of multiple fractures or severely reduced bone density at a young age.

Assessing the Risk of Fracture

Further evaluation is also indicated to estimate the actual fracture risk. Many factors contribute to the fracture risk in these patients (Table 5-3); these are discussed more thoroughly in Chapter 3. The most significant of these seem to be the magnitude of the bone mass deficit, the patient's age, a history of previous fragility fractures, and a propensity to fall from a standing posture. The bone mass deficit and the patient's age are easily assessed from readily available data. The history of previous fragility fractures can be approached initially by taking a careful history of back pain, serial measurements of standing height, and physical examination for dorsal kyphosis or vertebral point tenderness. More sensitive tests include lateral x-rays of the thoracic and lumbar spine[6] and morphometric x-ray absorptiometry.[7] Although many vertebral fractures are readily apparent on radiologic evaluation, more subtle

Table 5-3.	Risk Factors for Fragility Fractures
	Low bone mass
	Age ≥ 65 years
	Fracture after age 50 years
	Maternal history of fracture after age 50 years
	Low body weight (≤ 125 lb)
	Corticosteroid use
	Other secondary causes of osteoporosis

fractures may be detected only by careful morphometric analysis.[6,7] Although various criteria have been proposed, we recommend those listed in Table 5-4 for identification of a morphometric vertebral fracture.[6,7] The risk of falling can be assessed by ascertaining the history of falls within the past year, by evaluation of general health status and medication use, and by a thorough physical examination that includes evaluation of vision, stance stability, gait characteristics, and ability to rise from a chair. Risk factors for falling are shown in Table 5-5.[8,9]

Bone remodeling assessment can also be a valuable tool for the estimation of fracture risk. Bone remodeling consists of the resorption of old bone by osteo*clasts* and the formation of new bone by osteo*blasts* (Fig. 5-3). Tests for assessing the ongoing rate of osteoclastic bone resorption and osteoblastic bone formation are shown in Figure 5-4. Biomarker measurement has been demonstrated to pre-

Table 5-4.	Criteria for Identification of a Morphometric Vertebral Fracture

I. Semiquantitative diagnosis
  A. Grade 0: normal
  B. Grade 1: 20%–25% reduction in anterior, middle, or posterior height
  C. Grade 2: 25%–40% reduction in anterior, middle, or posterior height
  D. Grade 3: ≥ 40% reduction in anterior, middle, or posterior height
II. Quantitative diagnosis
  A. Prevalent vertebral fracture: 15% reduction in APR, MPR, or HPR compared with the mean value for that vertebra in a reference population. (APR = ratio of vertebral anterior height to posterior height, MPR = ratio of vertebral middle height to posterior height, HPR = ratio of vertebral posterior height to posterior height of adjacent vertebra)
  B. Incident vertebral fracture: 15% decrease in anterior, middle, or posterior height compared with previous radiograph of same vertebra

Data from Genant HK, Wu CY, Van Kuijk C, et al: Vertebral fracture assessment using a semiquantitative technique. J Bone Miner Res 8:1137–1148, 1993.

Table 5-5.   Risk Factors for Falling
Sedative use
Visual impairment
Abnormal gait
Abnormal balance
Neurologic disorders
Lower extremity disability
Unsafe home environment

Figure 5-3.   Bone remodeling is the ongoing process by which older bone is replaced by newer bone. The process begins with osteoclastic bone resorption. Osteoclasts are multinucleated cells that bind to the surface of bone and secrete enzymes, acid, and free radicals, which dissolve away bone mineral and collagen, leaving a resorption pit. Osteoblastic bone formation follows, as nearby osteoblasts are recruited to migrate in and fill the resorption pit with a bone-specific collagen, osteoid. If the concentrations of calcium and phosphorus in the extracellular fluids are adequate, calcium phosphate (hydroxyapatite) crystals precipitate in the newly laid osteoid to solidify and stabilize the newly formed bone tissue.

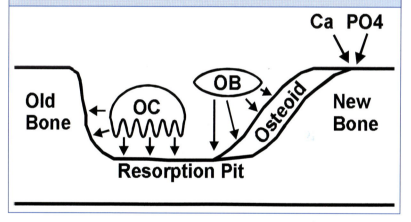

dict the likelihood of rapid bone loss[10,11] and the risk of fragility fractures developing[12,13] (Fig. 5-5). Because of the significant variability inherent in their measurements, it is best to collect specimens at the same time of day (second morning voided urine, fasting morning blood) on each occasion. Variation can also be reduced by averaging the result of two measurements or by pooling two samples on consecutive days.

Figure 5-4. Bone remodeling biomarkers. As bone is resorbed by osteoclasts, bone specific collagen fragments such as n-telopeptides, c-telopeptides, and pyridinoline cross-links are released into the circulation. As new bone is formed by osteoblasts, proteins such as bone-specific alkaline phosphatase and osteocalcin are secreted into the circulation. Measurements of these biomarkers can be used to assess the overall rate of skeletal remodeling.

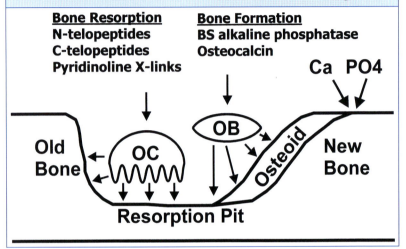

Figure 5-5. Bone remodeling biomarkers predict future hip fractures. In this prospective cohort study of 7598 healthy, elderly women (age > 75 years), a high baseline serum c-telopeptide (CTX) level significantly predicted the subsequent occurrence of hip fractures (odds ratio, 2.2; 95% CI; 1.3–3.6). The combination of a high serum CTX and a low hip BMD had greater predictive value (odds ratio, 4.8; 95% CI, 2.4–9.5) than either low hip BMD or high serum CTX alone. (Adapted from Garnero P, et al. Markers of bone resorption predict hip fracture in elderly women: the EPIDOS prospective study. J Bone Miner Res 11:1531–1538, 1996.)

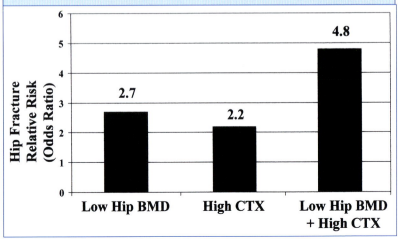

Key Points: Osteoporosis Evaluation

∽ Secondary disorders causing bone loss are present in approximately 30% of women and 64% of men who have osteoporosis.
∽ Patients who have a fragility fracture or low bone mass should have a complete history and physical examination and a limited number of key, cost-effective laboratory tests to identify any such underlying disorders.
∽ A complete fracture risk evaluation should also be conducted. In addition to bone densitometry testing, the most important elements of this include assessment of age, prior fragility fractures, and risk of falling.
∽ Bone remodeling biomarker measurement may also provide additional information in selected patients regarding the risk of future bone loss and the risk of future fractures.

References

1. Caplan GA, Scane AC, Francis RM: Pathogenesis of vertebral crush fractures in women. J R Soc Med 87:200–202, 1994.
2. Tannenbaum C, Clark J, Schwartzman K, et al: Yield of laboratory testing to identify secondary contributors to osteoporosis in otherwise healthy women. J Clin Endocrinol Metab 87:4431–4437, 2002.
3. Kelepouris N, Harper KD, Gannon F, et al: Severe osteoporosis in men. Ann Intern Med 123:452–460, 1995.
4. Harper KD, Weber TJ: Secondary osteoporosis: diagnostic considerations. Endocrinol Metab Clin North Am 27(2):325–348, 1998.
5. Orlic ZC, Raisz LG: Causes of secondary osteoporosis. J Clin Densitom 2:79–92, 1998.
6. Genant HK, Wu CY, Van Kuijk C, et al: Vertebral fracture assessment using a semi-quantitative technique. J Bone Miner Res 8:1137–1148, 1993.
7. Rea JA, Li J, Blake GM, et al: Visual assessment of vertebral deformity by x-ray absorptiometry: a highly predictive method to exclude vertebral deformity. Osteoporos Int 11(8):660–668, 2000.
8. Tinetti ME, Speechley M, Ginter SF: Risk factors for falls among elderly persons living in the community. N Engl J Med 319(26):1701–1707, 1998.
9. Grisso JA, Kelsey JL, Strom BL, et al: Risk factors for falls as a cause of hip fracture in women. N Engl J Med 324(19):1326–1331, 1991.
10. Rosen CJ, Chesnut III CH, Mallinak NJS: The predictive value of biochemical markers of bone turnover for bone mineral density in early postmenopausal women treated with hormone replacement of calcium supplementation. J Clin Endocrinol Metab 82:1904–1910, 1997.
11. Ross PD, Knowlton W: Rapid bone loss is associated with increased levels of biochemical markers. J Bone Miner Res 13:297–302, 1998.
12. Garnero P, Hausherr E, Chapuy M-C, et al: Markers of bone resorption predict hip fracture in elderly women: the EPIDOS prospective study. J Bone Miner Res 11:1531–1538, 1996.
13. Garnero P, Sornay-Rendu E, Claustrat B, et al: Biochemical markers of bone turnover, endogenous hormones and the risk of fractures in postmenopausal women: the OFELY study. J Bone Miner Res 15:1526–1536, 2000.

Prevention and Treatment of Osteoporosis: Nonpharmacologic

chapter

6

Carol Zapalowski, M.D., Ph.D. and Michael McDermott, M.D.

Nutrition affects bone quality in health and disease. Proper nutrition is critical for the cellular actions of osteocytes in maintaining bone density. Muscular function also depends on proper nutrition. Adequate muscular function is important in maintaining balance, preventing falls, and, thereby, preventing fractures. In addition, malnutrition can result in excessive thinness and lack of subcutaneous mass. Adequate soft tissue helps dissipate the force of a fall, which can also be important in decreasing fracture risk.

Two specific nutrients that are important in bone health, calcium and vitamin D, are discussed in this chapter. Magnesium, fluoride, phosphorus, and zinc are also important for their specific roles in bone composition but are not discussed in detail here.

Calcium

Calcium serves vital functions in all cells, acting as a second messenger and an essential cofactor. It is required for muscle contraction, hormone secretion, and cell division, as well as for bone mineralization. Calcium homeostasis is maintained by complex interactions that keep the extracellular fluid calcium concentration within a tight range. These homeostatic mechanisms regulate absorption, excretion, and redistribution of calcium between bone and other body compartments. The main hormones that affect calcium homeostasis are parathyroid hormone, calcitonin, and 1,25 dihydroxyvitamin D_3.[1,2]

The skeleton serves as a reservoir for the body's calcium, containing more than 99% of the body's calcium.[3] There is nearly constant remodeling of the skeleton; the osteoclastic bone resorption and osteoblastic bone formation are tightly coupled. Parathyroid hormone and other

45

hormones and activation factors, including 1,25 dihydroxyvitamin D_3, affect osteoclast and osteoblast function and are involved in skeletal calcium release and reaccumulation. In bone, calcium also provides structural strength. Calcium differs from most other nutrients in that the body contains a substantial store of it. This store far exceeds short-term needs for calcium and also serves a critical structural role. Because of the large stores of calcium, it takes a significant deficit to result in hypocalcemia, which would be recognized clinically as weakness, tetany, or arrhythmias. Before reaching the point of hypocalcemia, long-term calcium deficit manifests itself clinically as osteoporotic fracture. Even osteoporotic fracture does not occur until significant calcium stores have been lost. It has been shown in laboratory animals that bone mass will be sacrificed to preserve extracellular fluid calcium levels during periods of negative calcium balance.[2]

Calcium also serves as an antiresorptive agent, thereby preventing bone loss. Calcium intake can reduce age-related bone loss and improve bone accretion during growth.[2,3] Genetics, endogenous and exogenous estrogen, exercise, age-related differences in calcium absorption, medications, and dietary intake of calcium also affect bone retention of calcium and the risk for osteoporosis.

Calcium Requirements

Most experts would agree that adequate calcium intake is important for health at all life stages. There is less agreement regarding precise recommendations for appropriate calcium intake. Numerous studies have been done that look at calcium intake during growth and adulthood and in the aged.[4] Conflicting results have led to some scientific uncertainty, but several consensus groups have met to review the data and make recommendations. In 1997, the National Academy of Sciences reviewed the Recommended Dietary Allowances (RDAs) for calcium and thought that they were inadequate. At that time, the Dietary Reference Intakes (DRIs) were established for calcium and vitamin D.[5] Unlike the RDAs, which were meant to establish the minimal amount of a nutrient needed to be protected against possible nutrient deficiency, the DRIs were designed to reflect nutrient requirements on the basis of optimizing health in individuals and groups. Calcium recommendations were set at levels associated with maximum retention of body calcium, because it had been shown by that time that calcium and vitamin D could prevent bone loss and, in some populations, prevent fracture.

Calcium requirements vary throughout a person's lifetime. Requirements are greatest during puberty, when a significant proportion of one's peak bone mass is accumulated. There is evidence to suggest that the rate of bone acquisition during puberty is related to calcium intake. However, there is no evidence that accelerating the rate of accumulation during puberty results in a higher peak adult bone mass. Cross-sectional studies have shown that there is an association between lifelong calcium intake and peak adult bone mass. Therefore, one can reasonably assume that intake of calcium during the bone-forming years of childhood and young adulthood is important in the acquisition of optimal peak adult bone mass. The National Institutes of Health (NIH) consensus statement recommends 1200 to 1500 mg/day of elemental calcium for adolescents and young adults. The DRI at this age is 1300 mg/day.[4]

Women

Population studies in American girls and women suggest that calcium intake typically decreases to well below the NIH recommendation by the age of 11. Younger children are more likely than teens to have adequate calcium intake. Unfortunately, it is at the time that calcium intake falls off that girls enter puberty, and the hormonal milieu is optimal for acquisition of bone mass. Population surveys of girls and young women ages 12 to 19 years showed their typical calcium intake to be < 900 mg/day, only 60% of the NIH recommendation. This certainly raises concerns that these girls will be at risk for lower peak bone mass later in life.[6]

Bone density in women usually remains stable in early adulthood. Estrogen improves the efficiency of intestinal calcium absorption and decreases renal calcium excretion.[7] In addition, estrogen is an antiresorptive agent for bone. Because of estrogen's positive effects on calcium absorption from the gut and direct antiresorptive effects at the level of the osteoclast, the skeletal calcium requirements for this age group of women are typically met by their dietary intake. The NIH recommends 1000 mg/day of elemental calcium for adult women, and the DRI in this age group is 1200 mg of elemental calcium per day.

In contrast to prior recommendations, the new DRIs for calcium and vitamin D during pregnancy and lactation are not higher than the usual recommendation for age. During pregnancy and lactation, a fetus and infant require 7%–10% of a woman's total body calcium stores for their own development.[6] One might expect that unless a woman had adequate calcium intake to cover this loss during pregnancy and lactation, a net decrease in bone density would result. On the contrary, epidemiologic studies have shown that most women either maintain or increase bone mass during pregnancy and have a small decrease during lactation, which is reaccumulated shortly after resumption of menses. This may be due to an increase in physiologic conservation of calcium during pregnancy. Intestinal absorption of calcium is more efficient during pregnancy, and many women therefore begin lactating with a skeletal surplus of calcium. The NIH consensus statement recommends 1200–1500 mg/day of elemental calcium for pregnant and lactating women; the DRI is 1300 mg for women younger than 25 and 1000 mg of elemental calcium per day for women older than 25 years of age.[4]

During periods of estrogen deficiency, it is not uncommon for women to lose bone mass. Anorexia, hypogonadotropic amenorrhea, and drugs that block estrogen production, such as Depo-Provera and GnRH agonists, can all lead to periods of relative estrogen deficiency. Although data are lacking, during times of relative estrogen deficiency, it is prudent to recommend increased calcium consumption, similar to that recommended in postmenopausal women who are estrogen deficient.

Bone mass in women begins to fall with the drop in estrogen during menopause. Studies show that calcium and vitamin D alone cannot prevent this early menopausal bone loss, but it is possible that the magnitude of the loss is less. The benefits of calcium and vitamin D have been demonstrated clearly only in more elderly women. However, it is likely that women in perimenopause still need calcium and vitamin D to optimize bone health. The NIH consensus statement and the DRI recommend 1000 mg of elemental calcium per day for women 25–50 years of age. For women between 50 and 65 years of age (early postmenopausal), it is recommended by the NIH that 1500 mg of elemental calcium per day be consumed by those not on hormone replacement therapy and 1000 mg of elemental calcium per day for those on hormone replacement therapy. The DRI is 1200 mg for all women in this age group.

In the elderly, supplemental calcium has been shown to suppress biochemical markers of bone resorption and increase bone density at the spine, hip, and radius.[8] Intestinal calcium absorption is decreased in the elderly. This may be due to decreased vitamin D levels, interfering medications, or intrinsic decreased intestinal calcium absorption efficiency. Compounding the problem further, in both men and women older than 65 years of age, the typical calcium intake is only 600 mg/day.[6]

Because of the higher prevalence of osteoporosis and fractures in the elderly, relatively smaller and shorter studies can show differences with various interventions, including calcium and vitamin D, whereas definitive proof of cause and effect is difficult to ascertain in younger populations. The fracture incidence in younger age groups is very low, and the size and length of a study required to show a statistical difference between treated and untreated populations would be prohibitive.

Therefore, most data with all interventions for osteoporosis, both phar-macologic and nonpharmacologic, has been accumulated in older patient populations.

In an often-cited study by Chapuy et al[9] (Fig. 6–1), there was a sig-nificant loss in bone mass of 3% per year at the femur in women with a calcium intake averaging 514 mg/day. The bone loss was prevented with calcium and vitamin D supplementation. The study also showed a significant reduction in hip fracture risk at 18 months. Other studies by Chevalley et al,[10] Dawson-Hughes et al,[11,12] and Recker et al[13] also showed that calcium supplementation reduced age-related bone loss and decreased vertebral fracture incidence. The calcium intakes in these three studies approximated 1300–1500 mg/day.

There have also been studies that have shown no effect of calcium on bone density and fracture. In a meta-analysis by Shea,[14] the authors conclude that there is a small, but statistically significant, effect of cal-cium supplementation on bone loss in postmenopausal women. Supplementation with calcium has been shown to increase BMD at both the spine and the hip. A smaller number of studies were reviewed that looked at the effect of calcium supplementation on fracture rate. The authors concluded that the five studies that they included in the

Figure 6-1. In a randomized controlled trial, 3270 healthy elderly women were given either calcium, 1200 mg/day and cholecalciferol D, 800 IU/day or placebo. The figure shows the number of hip fractures and nonvertebral frac-tures in these women, whose mean age was 84 years. There was a statistically significant reduction in fractures of the hip, as well as in nonvertebral frac-tures. (Adapted from Chapuy M et al. Vitamin D3 and calcium to prevent hip fractures in elderly women. N Engl J Med 327:1637–1642, 1992.)

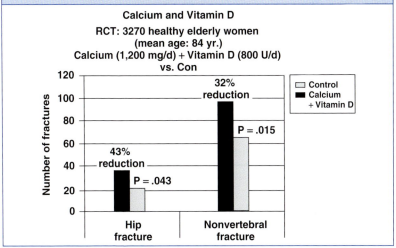

meta-analysis suggested a potentially important reduction in vertebral fractures and a smaller reduction in the risk of nonvertebral fractures. For both vertebral and nonvertebral fractures, the effect of calcium was consistent across trials but was not statistically significant. This meta-analysis is an excellent review of the studies done to date.

In response to these and other studies, the NIH consensus conference has recommended a calcium intake of 1500 mg/day in men and women older than age 65. The DRI in this age group is 1200 mg/day.

Men

There are fewer data correlating calcium intake and fracture risk in men. The effect of calcium alone on bone mass has not been evaluated in men. There have been two studies looking at the effect of calcium and vitamin D on the rates of bone loss in men. Dawson-Hughes et al[12] found that in older men with usual calcium intakes of approximately 750 mg/day, supplementation with 500 mg of calcium and 700 IU vitamin D significantly reduced bone loss from the spine, femoral neck, and total body during the first year and significantly reduced bone loss from the total body in years 2 and 3. Orwoll et al[15] found no significant effect on the rates of bone loss in men who had usual calcium intakes of about 1200 mg/day. In this study, men were given 1000 mg of calcium and 800 IU vitamin D. The NIH recommendation for men aged 25–65 is 1000 mg/day of elemental calcium, and the DRI is 1000 to 1200 mg/day. In men older than age 65, the NIH recommends 1500 mg, and the DRI is 1200 mg of elemental calcium per day.[4,5]

Optimal Calcium Requirements

Calcium can be obtained from dietary sources and/or supplementation. The two sources should be combined when calculating the total daily calcium intake. Table 6-1 summarizes the recommendations for calcium intake made by the NIH Consensus Development Conference in 1994[4] and the DRI implemented by the National Academy of Sciences in 1997.[5]

Sources of Calcium: Dietary Calcium

The optimal way for a person to achieve the recommended intake of calcium is through dietary sources. Calcium-fortified foods and calcium supplements can be added to make up the balance. Dairy products are excellent sources of calcium. Most dairy products contain approximately 300 mg of elemental calcium per serving. In the United States, milk and some other dairy products are supplemented with vitamin D as well. Some vegetables and fish (usually when the bones are consumed) are also good sources of calcium. Kale and broccoli are good sources of calcium. A 2½ cup serving of either contains 300 mg of calcium. A diet without dairy products or calcium-rich or -enriched foods usually provides only about 200–300 mg of calcium per day.[6]

Certain foods contain components that can result in decreased calcium absorption or increased calcium excretion. Foods high in oxalate and phytate can impair calcium absorption by binding to calcium in the gut. Foods high in oxalate include spinach and rhubarb. Foods high in phytate include legumes such as navy beans, peas, pinto beans, and wheat bran. The calcium in legumes has only half the bioavailability of the calcium in milk, whereas the calcium of spinach and rhubarb is nearly totally unavailable. Foods that contain oxalate and phytate will interfere with calcium absorption from other food sources only during meals in which they are consumed and not with the absorption of calcium taken at other times throughout the day. Dietary fiber, except for wheat bran, does not interfere with calcium absorption. There has been some suggestion that caffeine interferes with calcium absorption. If there

Table 6-1.	Recommendations for Optimal Calcium Intake*	
Age Group	NIH Optimal Daily Intake of Calcium (mg)	NAS Optimal Daily Intake of Calcium (mg)
Infants		
Birth–6 m.	400 mg	210 mg
6 m–1 y	600 mg	270 mg
Children		
1–5 y	800 mg	500 mg (1–3 y), 800 mg (4–5 y)
6–10 y	800–1200 mg	800 mg (6–8 y), 1300 mg (8–10 y)
Adolescents/young adults		
11–24 y	1200–1500 mg	1000–1300 mg
Men		
25–65 y	1000 mg	1000–1200 mg
>65 y	1500 mg	1200 mg
Women		
25–50 y	1000 mg	1000 mg
>50 y (postmenopausal):		
On estrogens	1000 mg	1200 mg
Not on estrogens	1500 mg	1200 mg
>65 years	1500 mg	1200 mg
Pregnant and nursing	1200–1500 mg	1300 mg (≤18 y), 1000 mg (>18 y)

*Adapted from the NIH Consensus Development Conference Statement on Optimal Calcium Intake, 1994[4] and Dietary Reference Intakes from the National Academy of Sciences, 1997.[5]

*Total calcium is the sum of calcium obtained from dietary sources and supplementation.

is an effect of caffeine, it is small. Diets high in animal protein and sodium can increase calcium excretion in the urine, making daily requirements of calcium intake higher.[4,6,16,17]

Calcium-fortified products are available. These include fortified juices, fruit drinks, breads, and cereals, among others.

Sources of Calcium: Calcium Supplements

Numerous calcium preparations are available for supplementation of dietary intake (Table 6-2). The most common of these are calcium carbonate and calcium citrate. Less common preparations include calcium gluconate and calcium lactate. The labels can be very confusing, and it is important for patients to check the labels carefully, because frequently the amounts of calcium and vitamin D stated in the list of ingredients are for more than one tablet or capsule.

Table 6-2.	Examples of Common Calcium Preparations	
Preparation	**Elemental Calcium per Tablet (mg)**	**Vitamin D in Preparations Supplemented with Vitamin D* (in IU per Tablet)**
Calcium carbonate		
Caltrate	600 mg	200 IU
Oscal	500 mg	200 IU
Viactiv	500 mg	100 IU
Tums**	200 mg	0 IU
Tums EX**	300 mg	0 IU
Tums Ultra**	400 mg	0 IU
Tums 500**	500 mg	0 IU
Nature Made	500 mg	200 IU
Nature Made	600 mg	200 IU
Maalox†	222 mg	0 IU
Rolaids†	250 mg	0 IU
Calcium citrate		
Citracal‡	200 mg	0 IU
Citracal‡	250 mg	62.5 IU
Citracal‡	315 mg	200 IU
Multiple vitamins		
Women's One-a-Day	450 mg	400 IU
Centrum Silver	200 mg	400 IU

*Many calcium supplements are formulated both as a preparation with vitamin D and as a preparation without vitamin D.
**On the Tums bottles, both the full weight of two pills and a table with mg of elemental calcium for two tablets are given. For example, Tums EX is listed as 600 mg of elemental calcium for two tablets, with a total weight of 1500 mg of calcium carbonate in two pills.
†Both Maalox and Rolaids are listed as the full weight of calcium carbonate in two tablets on the outside label. For Maalox, the full weight of one tablet is listed as 600 mg, and for Rolaids, the full weight of the one tablet is listed as 675 mg.
‡All the Citracal preparations are listed as the amount for two pills on the label.

The recommended daily allowance for calcium is based on the amount of elemental calcium in a food or supplement. The various calcium salts have different percentages of elemental calcium on the basis of their chemical formulas. Calcium citrate is 18% calcium by weight, and calcium carbonate is 40% calcium by weight. For example, a 600-mg tablet of calcium carbonate contains 240 mg of elemental calcium, and a 950-mg tablet of calcium citrate contains 200 mg of calcium. It is important for patients to look at the amount of elemental calcium in each preparation, rather than the total weight of that same preparation. In addition, it is important to discuss with patients that the amount of calcium in a preparation stated on the front label often is for two or more tablets. It is important for them to check the label on the back to be sure of what they are getting in each pill.

Calcium preparations from unrefined oyster shells, bone meal, or dolomite should be avoided, because lead and mercury contamination has been found in some lots of these products.[4]

Timing of Calcium Intake and Absorption

The absorbability of calcium is affected by the presence or absence of a meal and the size of the calcium load. Absorption of calcium is most efficient at doses of 500 mg or less. Therefore, calcium supplements or calcium-rich foods should be taken in doses of 500 mg or less, in divided doses throughout the day.[18]

In general, calcium carbonate is better absorbed when taken with food than on an empty stomach. This is likely due to increased gastric acid production with a meal. This effect is especially important for people with reduced gastric acid production. Because the prevalence of achlorhydria increases with age, this may contribute to the decreased age-related calcium absorption efficiency. Calcium carbonate should be taken with meals. Calcium citrate can be taken with meals or on an empty stomach.

In at least one study, it has been shown that a dose of calcium at bedtime reduces the nighttime rise in parathyroid hormone. It is not known whether this is beneficial to bone physiology.

Calcium Losses

Calcium can be lost through the feces, urine, and the skin (sweat and sloughed skin cells). Fecal calcium losses can be quite high, as high as 90% of ingested calcium, especially at higher calcium intakes. Fecal calcium losses are mainly from unabsorbed dietary calcium but can also be from digestive excretions and sloughed intestinal cells. At low calcium intakes, a much lower percentage of the excreted calcium is from dietary sources, because there is greater absorption efficiency when lower amounts of calcium are ingested. Loss of calcium through sweat has not been well characterized but is thought to be approximately 30% of normal urinary losses. During periods of excessive sweat loss (i.e., periods of strenuous exercise or exertion), dermal calcium losses can be significantly higher.[3]

High sodium intake increases urinary calcium excretion.[16,17] High-sodium diets lead to increased sodium excretion and with it an obligatory loss of urinary calcium. This is because of the solvent drag effect of sodium on calcium. High-protein diets increase calcium absorption from the gut but also increase obligatory calcium loss through the urine.[3,18] Caffeine may affect calcium absorption and possibly increase calcium excretion, but the effect is relatively minor.[6]

Side Effects from Calcium Supplements

Calcium preparations may cause side effects, such as constipation or flatulence. Sometimes, switching from one preparation to another can be beneficial in this regard. Keeping well hydrated and increasing fiber intake can be helpful as well.

Calcium Interferes with Iron Absorption

Calcium can interfere with iron absorption.[4] This is an important consideration for calcium taken with meals or for patients taking iron supplements.

Vitamin D

Effect of Vitamin D on Bone Mineral Density and Fracture

Many studies have looked at the effect of vitamin D on BMD and fracture rate. These are described in detail in a meta-analysis by Papadimitropoulos et al.[19] The authors of this meta-analysis concluded that vitamin D improves bone density and decreases vertebral fractures, as well as possibly having an effect on the risk of nonvertebral fractures. Bone mineral density increases have been seen at both the spine and the femoral neck.[12,20] The current data do not distinguish between the relative effects of vitamin D_3 and hydroxylated vitamin D. Most studies looking at the effect of vitamin D on fracture risk were done with supplemental calcium as well, and therefore it is not clear whether vitamin D has effects on bone metabolism by itself, or whether the effects of vitamin D are seen only in the presence of supplemental calcium.

1,25 Dihydroxyvitamin D_3 increases intestinal absorption of calcium (Fig. 6-2). Vitamin D is also involved in intestinal phosphate transport. The first described clinical use of vitamin D was the cure of rickets. It has been shown that intravenous infusion of calcium into vitamin D–deficient rats will cure rickets in the absence of coadministered vitamin D, suggesting that the effect of vitamin D on rickets is predominantly an increase in intestinal calcium and phosphorus absorption rather than a direct effect of vitamin D on bone formation. 1,25 Dihydroxyvitamin D_3 has actually been shown to have an effect on osteoclasts to increase bone mineral resorption, which suggests that the main physiologic purpose of 1,25 dihydroxyvitamin D is to maintain extracellular calcium in the normal range. Vitamin D also has effects on osteoblasts, although these effects have been less well characterized.[21,22]

The two parent forms of vitamin D are ergocalciferol (vitamin D_2) and cholecalciferol (vitamin D_3). Ergocalciferol is used as a vitamin D supplement. Cholecalciferol is the natural form of the vitamin and is produced by irradiation of its precursor, 7-dehydrocholesterol (provitamin D_3). Near-ultraviolet frequency light causes conversion of provitamin D_3 to vitamin D_3 in the epidermal layer of the skin. Doses of cholecalciferol and ergocalciferol are usually expressed in international units (IU). Forty international units of cholecalciferol are equal to 1 µg of

Figure 6-2. Vitamin D is synthesized in the skin and obtained from the diet. It undergoes hydroxylations in both the liver and the kidney to form 1,25 dihydroxyvitamin D_3, the active form of the vitamin. 1,25 Dihydroxyvitamin D_3 has direct effects on bone in addition to its major effect of increasing gut absorption of calcium.

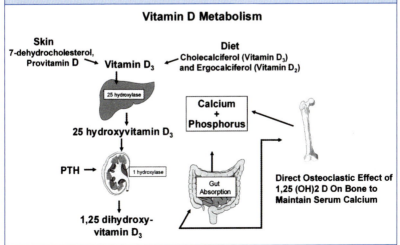

Vitamin D Metabolism

cholecalciferol. These units are used interchangeably in many publications and formulations of vitamin D. Calciferol refers to both of these compounds, ergocalciferol and cholecalciferol. In technical terms, vitamin D is not a vitamin, because it can be produced by the body. With enough exposure to sunlight, there can be adequate synthesis of vitamin D.[21,22]

Vitamin D can come from dietary sources. Few foods naturally contain significant amounts of vitamin D. Fish oil and egg yolks are two such foods. Dairy products contain insignificant amounts of vitamin D. However, in the United States, the Food and Drug Administration requires that each quart of milk have 10 μg (400 IU) of vitamin D added. Most multiple vitamins contain 400 IU of vitamin D.[6]

Both vitamin D_3 produced in the skin and vitamin D_3 from dietary sources and supplementation must undergo hydroxylation to produce the biologically active form, 1,25 dihydroxyvitamin D_3. The first hydroxylation occurs in the liver. Vitamin D_3 is hydroxylated to form 25 hydroxyvitamin D_3 in the liver. This is the main storage form of the molecule. A 25 hydroxyvitamin D_3 level is the single best laboratory test of overall vitamin D status. In the kidney, 25 hydroxyvitamin D_3 is converted to 1,25 dihydroxyvitamin D_3, the biologically active form.[21]

Patients with kidney disease can have vitamin D deficiency because of the inability to hydroxylate vitamin D_3 to its active form. In addition, medications that increase catabolism to vitamin D can result in vitamin D deficiency. The most notable medications are the anticonvulsants, phenobarbital and phenytoin, which increase catabolism of vitamin D in the liver.

The DRI for vitamin D is 400 IU per day for adults 50 to 70 years of age and 600 IU for adults older than 70 years of age. Many elderly patients require higher doses to maintain bone health.

Many calcium preparations contain vitamin D. The net total of vitamin D from a multivitamin and calcium/vitamin D supplement should equal 400 to 800 IU per day.

Vitamin D Deficiency

Vitamin D deficiency results in rickets in children. In adults, severe vitamin D deficiency may be seen as frank osteomalacia. Oftentimes, vitamin D insufficiency or deficiency results in secondary hyperparathyroidism (Fig. 6-3), bone loss, and an increased fracture risk.[22]

There is a significant amount of data to suggest a high prevalence of vitamin D deficiency in the elderly. Vitamin D deficiency can be related to a low intake of vitamin D, both dietary and as a supplement, and inadequate sunlight exposure. In elderly patients, there is decreased

Figure 6-3. Vitamin D deficiency is common throughout the world. In patients with malabsorption, vitamin D deficiency, or a calcium-poor diet, the calcium level is decreased slightly, and the serum parathyroid hormone level is increased as a secondary response. The levels of both calcium and parathyroid hormone can remain within the normal range. The increase in parathyroid hormone results in increased osteoclastic activity, increased bone resorption, and associated bone loss.

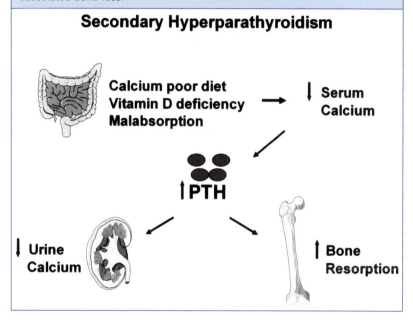

Secondary Hyperparathyroidism

conversion of provitamin D_3 to vitamin D_3 in the skin. In addition, elderly people are less likely to get adequate sunlight.

The use of sunscreen prevents the conversion of provitamin D_3 to vitamin D_3 in the skin and can contribute to vitamin D deficiency as well. 25 Hydroxyvitamin D_3 levels fluctuate with the season, are lower in the winter. Low vitamin D_3 levels are associated with secondary hyperparathyroidism and lower bone mass in the elderly.[20,22]

A person with osteoporosis might be suspected to be vitamin D deficient if his or her laboratory examination reveals a low 24-hour urinary calcium, low serum calcium, low serum phosphate, elevated serum alkaline phosphatase, elevated bone-specific alkaline phosphatase, or a urinary marker of bone resorption such as an N-telopeptide (NTx) that is elevated without other reason.

Inadequate vitamin D levels are more common than has been previously appreciated. Multiple studies have been done looking at the prevalence of vitamin D deficiency. It is not uncommon to see the prevalence of vitamin D insufficiency be > 25% in these studies, and it has been as high as 70% in studies done in northern latitudes in the winter.[23–25] If vitamin D deficiency is suspected, a serum 25 hydroxy-vitamin D level should be ordered. One might argue that because the prevalence of vitamin D deficiency is high, even in areas high in sunlight, a 25 hydroxyvitamin D level should be measured in all patients with osteoporosis. The cost-effectiveness of measuring a vitamin D level in the workup of osteoporosis has not been adequately evaluated.

Although nutritional vitamin D deficiency is common, other etiologies of vitamin D deficiency should always be considered, if clinically indicated. These include a lack of ultraviolet radiation exposure (being elderly, low sunlight exposure, and dark-skinned individuals), chronic renal insufficiency or renal failure, partial gastrectomy, intestinal malabsorption, chronic liver disease, and the use of anticonvulsant medications.[20,22]

The normal range for 25 hydroxyvitamin D in most laboratories is approximately 8–57 ng/mL. However, patients with levels of 25 hydroxyvitamin D between 8 and 25 ng/mL are likely vitamin D insufficient, and a level between 20 and 57 ng/mL is a more appropriate target level. Vitamin D levels < 20–25 ng/mL have been shown to be associated with secondary hyperparathyroidism, which may result in bone loss over time.

Excessive Vitamin D and Calcium Intake

The upper acceptable limit of calcium intake recommended by the RDI is 2500 mg/day. Over this amount, it is suggested that there might be an increase in the incidence of nephrolithiasis.

It is possible to become vitamin D intoxicated with excess doses of vitamin D. The upper acceptable limit of vitamin D intake as established by the RDI is 2000 IU/day. Excessive vitamin D ingestion can result in toxicity, manifested by hypercalcemia, hypercalciuria, bone resorption, bone loss, and renal functional impairment. The usual recommended dose of vitamin D_3 is 400–800 IU/day.[5] Although the RDI is 400 IU, an elderly patient may require 800 IU or more per day to keep his or her serum 25 hydroxyvitamin D levels > 20–25 ng/mL. Studies have been done using 50,000 IU per month and 100,000 to 300,000 IU by mouth or injection every 4 months to 1 year, and in these studies, there was no evidence of hypercalcemia. There have been case reports of hypercalcemia when doses of > 2000 IU/day of vitamin D_3 are used, but a 20-week dosing study with the highest dose being 10,000 IU/day of vitamin D_3 did not cause hypercalcemia in any of the groups.[26] Unfortunately, the occurrence of vitamin D intoxication is unpredictable, and patients on higher dosing regimens should be periodically monitored.

Conclusions Regarding Calcium and Vitamin D Nutrition

Optimal bone health requires adequate calcium and vitamin D. Current statistics suggest that calcium and vitamin D intake is below recommended levels in most individuals. It is important that education regarding calcium and vitamin D intake start in the pediatric age group and continue throughout life.

Exercise

Regular physical activity has wide-ranging health benefits for individuals of all ages, including important effects on bone health. It has been shown that physical activity early in life contributes to the development of a higher peak bone mass. Physical loading of bone is necessary for normal growth, development, and maintenance of the skeleton. Observational trials suggest that physical activity can reduce the risk for fracture in older individuals, although the value of exercise as an intervention for the prevention of postmenopausal bone loss is more controversial.

Physical activity benefits skeletal structure and strength. Wolff's law states that a stress or mechanical loading applied to the bone by muscles and tendons has a direct effect on bone formation and remodeling.[27] Various activities affect different parts of the skeleton differently, depending on the patterns of physical loading on specific bones. Physical activity variations include type, frequency, duration, intensity, and age of onset. An exercise must overload bone to stimulate it[28] (i.e., to increase bone density and/or bone strength and quality).

Studies in this area are difficult for several reasons. Compliance with prescribed exercise regimens has been a problem. Another issue is that physical fitness of the control group at baseline differs from study to study, and therefore the degree of change may vary. Trials of exercise intervention are more likely to show an effect in very inactive adults. Last, the rate of the response of bone to an exercise regimen is slower than for other physiologic interventions, and therefore studies must be continued for longer durations of time. Randomized controlled trials large enough and long enough to provide definitive answers to important questions, most specifically the effect of exercise on fracture rate, are not available and possibly never will be. Therefore, recommendations must be made from conclusions drawn from shorter-term trials.

It has been shown repeatedly in population studies that elite athletes have higher bone mass than nonathletes. The conclusion has been drawn from this that physical activity is beneficial to bone, but it may be that the individuals who choose to exercise may have predisposing skeletal characteristics that influenced their choice and ability to maintain an advanced level of physical activity. With the studies done so far, it is impossible to separate the effect of predisposing skeletal characteristics from the influence of exercise on bone quality.

Variations in the bone density response to different sports and activities reflect different and specific loading patterns of each sport on the skeleton. Studies with squash and tennis players show that a difference in bone density exists between playing and nonplaying arms, with the playing forearm having a higher bone density.[29] Sports that have similar influences bilaterally do not show such a difference. For example, runners and gymnasts have similar bone densities in both hips. A study by Beshgetoor[30] compared bone density in master cyclists, runners, and controls with a mean age of 50 years who exercise regularly but noncompetitively. In runners, BMD of the lumbar spine remained stable, but BMD of the lumbar spine went down in the cyclists and controls.

If an exercise program is expected to increase bone density at a specific site, it must load the bones at that site. Methods of bone overload include frequency, duration, and intensity of exercise. Of these, bone seems to be most influenced by exercise intensity. Exercises resulting in high impact have been shown to stimulate bone mass accretion, particularly at the hip. An example of this is the difference between gymnasts and runners. During a training session, gymnasts increase bone mass, whereas runners do not. This is because runners experience forces at the ground of >12 times body weight, whereas these body forces are only three to five times body weight in gymnasts. An increase in bone density is not seen in runners with training, despite the fact that the activity is high in repetitions.[28,31,32]

A strong positive relationship between body mass and BMD or content has been shown. This is likely because of increased gravitational forces on bone. Weight loss may be a risk factor for loss of bone mass. Women aged 44–50 years on a dietary intervention who lost an average of 3.2±4.7 kg over 18 months were observed to lose more bone mass at the hip and spine than control subjects who did not lose weight.[33]

Muscle forces impart considerable physical loads on bone. Hip, spine, whole-body, and tibial BMDs have all been positively correlated with back, bicep, quadricep, and grip strength. Back extensor muscle mass and strength have been shown to be one of the strongest predictors of BMD at many sites, including the spine and the hip.[28]

The removal of regular weight-bearing activity generates an adaptive skeletal response in both humans and animals, resulting in generalized bone loss. Human models of disuse osteoporosis, including bed rest, spinal cord injury, and exposure to the weightlessness of space travel, result in negative calcium balance, alterations in biochemical markers of bone turnover, and loss of bone mineral. This response is site specific, that is, the loss occurs predominantly in the bones that are unloaded.[34] Similarly, athletes who discontinue training and athletes during the off-season consistently show a decreased BMD at the specific sites that were initially increased by their exercise.[35]

Children and Young Adults

Osteoporosis can result from inadequate bone mass accrual during childhood and adolescence, lack of maintenance of bone mass during adulthood, or a combination of both. Peak adult bone mass, the amount of bone mass achieved at the conclusion of growth, is an important predictor of future osteoporosis.

Studies in children and adolescents, for the most part, show a significant association between physical activity and bone density at the total body, hip, spine, and forearm. Increased activity during childhood and adolescence results in an increased peak adult bone mass.[36] It is not known whether physical activity during childhood will benefit bone strength and quality, as well as bone density, throughout one's life. Whether the attainment of a normal peak adult bone mass prevents fractures later in life has not been definitively established, although this would make intuitive sense. Again, because of the length of the study required to establish this relationship, the definitive answer is likely not going to be established in the near future.

Most of the sports that children participate in are impact-type sports, such as baseball, basketball, soccer, and gymnastics. Impact sports have been shown to be effective at increasing bone density before, during, and after puberty. Studies are conflicting as to whether exercise is most important prepubertally or during puberty for the acquisition of the highest bone mass possible.[29,36–41] Swimming and resistance strength training have been shown to be of little benefit to bone density acquisition, but no studies regarding bone strength and quality with nonimpact exercises have been done to date.

Adult Women, Premenopausal and Postmenopausal

Most studies on exercise have been done in postmenopausal women.[28,42–46] Impact and strength exercises in postmenopausal women have been shown to increase BMD at both the hip and the spine.[47–53] Studies have also shown, although not consistently, that women who exercise have a reduction in the number of fractures and a stabilization of their height.[49,54,55] No long-term prospective randomized controlled trials of physical activity exploring fracture outcomes have been done.

Studies done in early postmenopausal women are few in number and conflicting. Some studies show prevention of bone loss with exercise in the early postmenopausal time frame, and others show no effect. More data will need to be collected before conclusions are made regarding early postmenopausal prevention of bone loss with exercise.[56]

It has been concluded in several studies that continued training is likely required to maintain the musculoskeletal benefit from exercise.[57,58] The studies have shown that when training is discontinued, bone density decreases back toward baseline.

In many small studies, high-impact exercises have been shown to increase BMD, whereas lower impact exercises have not been shown to improve BMD in postmenopausal women. A large population study by Feskanich et al[59] evaluated the incidence of hip fractures in the 61,200 postmenopausal women aged 40 to 77 in the Nurses Health Study cohort. These women were stratified into various activity levels and followed for 12 years. The study was controlled for use of postmenopausal hormones, body mass index, smoking, and dietary intakes. The risk of hip fracture was lowered by 6% for each increase of 3 metabolic-equivalent hours per week of activity (equivalent to 1 hour per week of walking at an average pace). Active women with at least 24 metabolic-equivalent hours per week had a 55% lower risk of hip fracture than sedentary women with less than 3 metabolic-equivalent hours per week. The risk of hip fracture decreased linearly with an increasing level of activity among women not taking postmenopausal hormones but not among women taking hormones. More time spent standing was also independently associated with a lower risk for fracture. This study corroborated and elaborated on data by Puntila et al,[60] which showed an increase in BMD in active postmenopausal women compared with sedentary individuals.

Men

Few studies on exercise and bone density have been done in men. A meta-analysis by Kelley et al[61] concluded that site-specific exercise may likely improve and maintain BMD at the spine and hip, but the data were limited, and the changes seen were small. In a subsequent study by Huuskonen et al,[62] 140 men were followed for 4 years and did not show an effect of regular aerobic activity on femoral neck BMD. In a larger study by Kujala et al,[63] involving 3262 men older than age 44, an inverse relationship between baseline physical activity and future fracture risk was seen among men, with a relative risk for fracture of 0.38

in men participating in vigorous physical activity compared with sedentary men. In a population study that likely reflects a cross-section of the U.S. male population, Mussolino et al[64] reported BMD results from 4254 men who participated in the NHANES III. They concluded that jogging was associated with a higher BMD.

Fall Prevention and Physical Activity

It seems intuitively obvious that because exercise is involved in the maintenance of strength, flexibility, and balance, exercise would be directly related to falls in the elderly. However, long-term interventions proving this hypothesis are inconsistent.[28,65] Muscle weakness by itself is an independent risk factor for hip fracture,[66] and it is well known that exercise is directly related to muscle strength. Exercise is also related to flexibility and balance, and thereby could be important in the prevention of falls by this mechanism.[66,67] Most hip and Colles' fractures occur with falls, and it is likely that a significant percentage of vertebral fractures are also related to falls.[28]

Conclusions Regarding Exercise

It is likely that exercise is involved in the acquisition of normal peak adult bone mass and that continued exercise is necessary to maintain bone mass gained during childhood and adolescence. In some studies, increases in bone density and decreases in fracture risk have been seen with exercise. Exercise has the added benefit of improving strength, flexibility, and balance, and thereby may be related to the number of falls and fractures in the elderly. In many cases, further randomized controlled trials are required to make definitive conclusions.

Habit Alteration

Smoking has been identified as a risk factor for low bone mass and for the occurrence of fragility fractures.[68,69] Alcohol abuse has also been reported to be a risk factor for low bone mass and an increased fracture risk,[70,71] particularly in men.[72] The mechanisms for the effects of these habits likely relate to nutritional issues, lower body mass, less exercise, and reduced levels of gonadal steroids that may be associated with tobacco and alcohol abuse. Although discontinuation of these habits has not been prospectively shown to reverse their adverse skeletal effects, it would seem prudent and cost-effective to recommend smoking cessation and a reduction or cessation of alcohol intake for all patients of concern.

Fall Prevention

Fall prevention should also be given high priority in patients who have an increased fracture risk. Falls have been clearly shown to precede most hip fractures and nearly all wrist fractures. Risk factors for falls have been clearly identified and include sedative use, vision impairment, neurologic disorders, lower extremity disability, and other abnormalities of balance and gait.[73,74] Falls may also result from obstacles or hazards in the home that pose a risk for stumbling or slipping. Identification of these conditions with a careful history, physical examination, and home environment study and subsequent correction of those that can be modified can significantly reduce the fall risk of individuals at high risk for fractures (Fig. 6-4).[75–78] Hip protectors have also been developed to pad the hip and thereby disperse the impact energy of a fall. A randomized controlled trial examining the use of hip protectors in 1801 ambulatory but frail elderly adults reported a 60% reduction (relative hazard, 0.4; 95% CI, 0.2–0.8) in the incidence of hip fractures in the hip protector group compared with the controls (Fig. 6-5). We believe that greater attention

Figure 6-4. Fall prevention strategies lower risks of falling and hip fracture in nursing home residents. In this randomized controlled trial (RCT) of 402 nursing home residents (median age, 83 years), 194 were randomly assigned to a multiple risk factor intervention strategy, and 208 were randomly assigned to usual care. In the intervention group, there was a 51% reduction (adjusted odds ratio, 0.49; 95% CI, 0.37–0.65) in the risk of falling and a 77% reduction (adjusted odds ratio, 0.23; 95% CI, 0.06–0.94) in the risk of fracturing a hip. (Adapted from Jensen J, Lundin-Olssen L, Nyberg L, et al. Fall and injury prevention in older people living in residential care facilities. Ann Intern Med 136:733–741, 2002.)

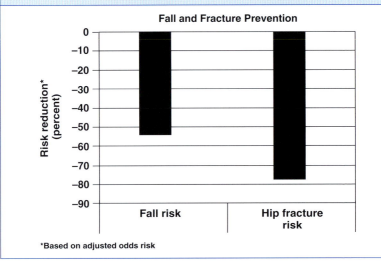

Fall and Fracture Prevention

*Based on adjusted odds risk

Figure 6-5. Hip protectors reduce the risk of hip fracture in elderly people. In this randomized controlled trial (RCT), 1801 elderly ambulatory but frail adults (mean age 82 years) were randomly assigned to wear hip protectors or to be in the control group. There was a 60% reduction (relative hazard, 0.4; 95% CI, 0.2–0.8; $P = 0.008$) in the risk of subsequent hip fractures in the group who wore hip protectors. (Adapted from Kannus P, Parkkari J, Niemi S, et al. Prevention of hip fracture in elderly people with use of a hip protector. N Engl J Med 343:1506–1513, 2000).

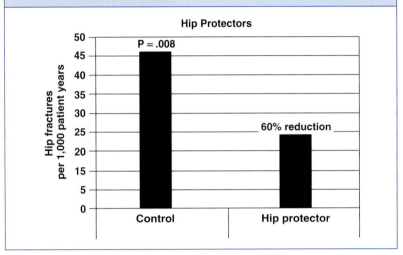

Key Points: Nonpharmacologic Treatment of Osteoporosis

- Nonpharmacologic treatment modalities are of significant value and should be implemented in all patients for whom treatment or prevention of osteoporosis is a goal.
- Adequate calcium and vitamin D nutrition is critical in the management of patients with osteoporosis. Failure to achieve adequate calcium and vitamin D intake and absorption leads to secondary hyperparathyroidism with resultant bone loss.
- Exercise improves bone mass and muscle strength, coordination, and balance. Exercise should be an integral part of all osteoporosis prevention and treatment plans.
- Individuals who have or who want to prevent osteoporosis should avoid smoking tobacco and should limit alcohol consumption.
- Fall risk evaluation and fall prevention measures are also key components of osteoporosis management strategies.

to preventing falls and the use of hip protectors can be a highly effective and cost-efficient fracture prevention strategy that is complementary to the nutrition, exercise, and medication interventions available to manage patients with osteoporosis.

References

1. Brown EM: Physiology and pathophysiology of the extracellular calcium-sensing receptor. Am J Med 106:238–253, 1999.
2. Brown EM: *Physiology of calcium metabolism*. In Becker KL (ed): Principles and Practice of Endocrinology and Metabolism. Philadelphia, Lippincott Williams & Wilkins, 2001.
3. Power ML, Heaney RP, Kalkwarf HJ, et al: The role of calcium in health and disease. Am J Obstet Gynecol 181(6):1560–1569, 1999.
4. NIH Consensus Statement Online: Optimal calcium intake. NIH Consensus Statement 12(4):1–31, 1994.
5. Institute of Medicine: Dietary Reference Intakes: Calcium, Phosphorus, Magnesium, Vitamin D, and Fluoride. Washington: National Academy Press, 1997.
6. Heaney RP: Nutrition and risk for osteoporosis. Osteoporosis 2(1):669–700, 2001.
7. Heaney RP, Recker RR, Stegman MR: Calcium absorption in women: relationships to calcium intake, estrogen status, and age. J Bone Miner Res 4:469–475, 1989.
8. Dawson Hughes B: The role of calcium in the treatment of osteoporosis. Osteoporosis 2(2):545–552, 2001.
9. Chapuy MC, Arlot ME, Duboeuf F, et al: Vitamin D3 and calcium to prevent hip fractures in elderly women. N Engl J Med 327:1637–1642, 1992.
10. Chevalley T, Rizzoli R, Nydegger V, et al: Effects on calcium supplements on femoral bone mineral density and vertebral fracture rate in vitamin-D-replete elderly patients. Osteoporos Int 4:245–252, 1994.
11. Dawson-Hughes B, Dallai GE, Krall EA, et al: A controlled trial of the effects of calcium supplementation on bone density in postmenopausal women. N Engl J Med 323:878–883, 1990.
12. Dawson-Hughes B, Harris SS, Krall EA, et al: Calcium and vitamin D supplementation on bone density in men and women 65 years of age or older. N Engl J Med 337:670–676, 1997.
13. Recker R, Hinders S, Davies KM, et al: Correcting calcium nutritional deficiency prevents spine fractures in elderly women. J Bone Miner Res 11:1961–1966, 1996.
14. Shea B, Wells G, Cranney A, et al and The Osteoporosis Methodology Group, The Osteoporosis Research Advisory Group: Meta-analysis of calcium supplementation for the prevention of postmenopausal osteoporosis. Endocrine Rev 23(4):552–559, 2002.
15. Orwoll ES, Oviatt SK, McClung MR, et al: The rate of bone mineral loss in normal men and the effects of calcium and cholecalciferol supplementation. Ann Intern Med 112:29–34, 1990.
16. Nordin BE, Need AG, Morris HA, et al: Sodium, calcium, and osteoporosis. In Burckhardt P, Heaney RP (ed). Serono Symposium Publication. Volume 85: Nutritional Aspects of Osteoporosis. New York, Raven Press, 1991, p 279.
17. Dawson-Hughes B, Fowler SE, Dalsky G, et al: Sodium excretion influences calcium homeostasis in elderly men and women. J Nutr 126:2107–2112, 1996.
18. Atkinson SA, Ward WE: Clinical nutrition: 2. The role of nutrition in the prevention and treatment of adult osteoporosis. CMAJ-JAMC 165(11):1511–1514, 2001.

19. Papadimitropoulos E, Wells G, Shea B, et al and The Osteoporosis Methodology Group, The Osteoporosis Research Advisory Group: VIII: Meta-analysis of the efficacy of vitamin D treatment in preventing osteoporosis in postmenopausal women. Endo Rev 23(4):560–569, 2002.
20. Reid IR: Vitamin D and its metabolites in the management of osteoporosis. Osteoporosis 2(2):553–575, 2001.
21. Clemens L, O'Riordan L: Vitamin D. In Kenneth I. Becker (ed.) Principles and Practice of Endocrinology and Metabolism, Philadelphia, Lippincott Williams & Wilkins, 2001.
22. Lips P: Vitamin D deficiency and secondary hyperparathyroidism in the elderly: consequences for bone loss and fractures and therapeutic implications. Endocr Rev 22:477–501, 2001.
23. Thomas MK, Lloyd-Jones DM, Thadhani RI, et al: Hypovitaminosis D in medical inpatients. N Engl J Med 338:777–783, 1998.
24. LeBoff MS, Kohlmeier L, Hurwitz S, et al: Occult vitamin D deficiency in postmenopausal US women with acute hip fracture. JAMA 281:1505–1511, 1999.
25. Outila TA, Karkkainen MU, Lamberg-Allardt CJ: Vitamin D status affects serum parathyroid hormone concentrations during winter in female adolescents: Associations with forearm bone mineral density. Am J Clin Nutr 74:206–210, 2001.
26. Heaney RP, Davies KM, Chen TC, et al: Human serum 25–hydroxycholecalciferol response to extended oral dosing with cholecalciferol. Am J Clin Nutr 77:204–210, 2003.
27. Chamay A, Tschantz P: Mechanical influences in bone remodeling. Experimental research on Wolff's law. J Biomech 5:173–180, 1972.
28. Beck BR, Shaw J, Snow CM: Physical activity and osteoporosis. Osteoporosis 2(1):701–720, 2001.
29. Kannus P, Haapasalo H, Sankelo M, et al: Effect of starting age of physical activity on bone mass in the dominant arm of tennis and squash players. Ann Intern Med 123: 27–31, 1995.
30. Beshgetoor D, Nichols JF, Rego I: Effect of training mode and calcium intake on bone mineral density in female master cyclists, runners, and non-athletes. Int J Sport Nutr Exerc Metab 10:290–301, 2000.
31. Taaffe DR, Robinson TL, Snow CM, et al: High-impact exercise promotes bone gain in well-trained female athletes. J Bone Miner Res 12:255–260, 1997.
32. LaRiviere J, Snow CM, Robinson TL: Bone mass changes in female competitive gymnasts over two seasons. Med Sci Sports Exerc 28:S131, 1996.
33. Salamone LM, Cauley JA, Black DM, et al: Effect of a lifestyle intervention on bone mineral density in premenopausal women: a randomized trial. Am J Clin Nutr 70(1):97–103, 1999.
34. Giangregorio L, Blimkie CJR: Skeletal adaptations to alterations in weight-bearing activity. A comparison of models of disuse osteoporosis. Sports Med 32(7):459–476, 2002.
35. Snow CM, Williams DP, LaRiviere J, et al: Bone gains and losses follow seasonal training and detraining in gymnasts. Calcif Tissue Int 69(1):7–12, 2001.
36. Vuori IM: Dose-response of physical activity and low back pain, osteoarthritis, and osteoporosis. Med Sci Sports Exercise 33(6):S551–S586, 2001.
37. Khan KM, Bennell KL, Hopper JL, et al: Self-reported ballet classes undertaken at age 10–12 years and hip bone mineral density in later life. Osteoporos Int 8:165–173, 1998.
38. Nordstrom P, Nordstrom G, Thorsen K, et al: Local bone mineral density, muscle strength, and exercise in adolescent boys: A comparative study of two groups with different muscle strength and exercise levels. Calcif Tissue Int 58:402–408, 1996.
39. Slemenda CW, Reister TK, Hui SL, et al: Influences on skeletal mineralization in children and adolescents: evidence for varying effects of sexual maturation and physical activity. J Pediatr 125:201–207, 1994.

40. Bailey DA, McKay HA, Mirwald RL, et al: A six-year longitudinal study of the rela-tionship of physical activity to bone mineral accrual in growing children: The University of Saskatchewan Bone Mineral Accrual Study. J Bone Miner Res 14:1672–1679, 1999.
41. Fuchs RK, Bauer JJ, Snow CM: Jumping improves hip and lumbar spine bone mass in prepubescent children: a randomized controlled trial. J Bone Miner Res 16(1):148–156, 2001.
42. Lin JT, Lane JM: Nonmedical management of osteoporosis. Curr Opin Rheumatol 14(4):441–446, 2002.
43. Layne JE, Nelson ME: The effects of progressive resistance training on bone density: a review. Med Sci Sports Exerc 31(1):25–30, 1999.
44. Bonaiuti D, Shea B, Lovine R, et al: Exercise for preventing and treating osteoporosis in postmenopausal women (Cochrane Review). In The Cochrane Library, Issue 1 Oxford, Update Software, 2003.
45. Kelley G: Aerobic exercise and lumbar spine bone mineral density in post-menopausal women: a meta-analysis. J Am Geriatr Soc 46:143–152, 1998.
46. Kelley G: Aerobic exercise and bone density at the hip in postmenopausal women: a meta-analysis. Prev Med 27:798–807, 1998.
47. Chien MY, Wu YT, Hsu AT, et al: Efficacy of a 24-week aerobic exercise program for osteopenic postmenopausal women. Calcif Tissue Int 67:443–448, 2000.
48. Snow CM, Shaw JM, Winter KM, et al: Long-term exercise using weighted vests pre-vents hip bone loss in postmenopausal women. J Gerontol 55A:M489–M491, 2000.
49. Walker M, Klentrous P, Chow R, et al: Longitudinal evaluation of supervised versus unsupervised exercise programs for the treatment of osteoporosis. Eur J Appl Physiol 83:349–355, 2000.
50. Wallace BA, Cumming RG: Systematic review of randomized trials of the effect of exercise on bone mass in pre-and postmenopausal women. Calcif Tissue Int 67:10–8, 2000.
51. Wolff I, Van Croonenborg JJ, Kemper HCG, et al: The effect of exercise training pro-grams on bone mass: a meta-analysis of published controlled trials in pre- and post-menopausal women. Osteoporos Int 9:1–12, 1999.
52. Berard A, Bravo G, Gauthier P: Meta-analysis of the effectiveness of physical activity for the prevention of bone loss in postmenopausal women. Osteoporos Int 7:331–337, 1997.
53. Kerr D, Ackland T, Maslen B, et al: Resistance training over 2 years increases bone mass in calcium-replete postmenopausal women. J Bone Miner Res 16(1):175–181, 2001.
54. Joakimsen RM, Magnus JH, Fonnebo V: Physical activity and predisposition for hip fractures: a review. Osteoporosis Int 7(6):503–513, 1997.
55. Sagiv M, Vogelaere PP, Soudry M, et al: Role of physical activity training in attenua-tion of height loss through aging. Gerontology 46:266–270, 2000.
56. Kemmler W, Engelke K, Lauber D, et al: Exercise effects on fitness and bone mineral density in early postmenopausal women: 1-year EFOPS results. Med Sci Sports Exerc 34(12):2115–2123, 2002.
57. Winter KM, Snow CM: Detraining reverses positive effects of exercise on the muscu-loskeletal system in premenopausal women. J Bone Miner Res 15:2495–2503, 2000.
58. Iwamoto J, Takeda T, Ichimura S: Effect of exercise training and detraining on bone mineral density in postmenopausal women with osteoporosis. J Orthop Sci 6:128–132, 2001.
59. Feskanich D, Willett W, Graham C: Walking and leisure-time activity and risk of hip fracture in postmenopausal women. JAMA 288:2300–2306, 2002.

60. Puntila E, Kroger H, Lakka T, et al: Leisure-time physical activity and rate of bone loss among peri- and postmenopausal women: a longitudinal study. Bone 29(5): 442–446, 2001.
61. Kelley GA, Kelly KS, Tran ZV: Exercise and bone mineral density in men: a meta-analysis. J Appl Physiol 88:1730–1736, 2000.
62. Huuskonen J, Vaisanen SB, Kroger H, et al: Regular physical exercise and bone mineral density: a four-year controlled randomized trial in middle-aged men. The DNASCO study. Osteoporos Int 12:349–355, 2001.
63. Kujala U, Kaprio MD, Jaakko MD, et al: Physical activity and osteoporotic hip fracture risk in men. Arch Intern Med 160(5):705–708, 2000.
64. Mussolino ME, Looker AC, Orwoll ES: Jogging and bone mineral density in men: Results from NHANES III. Am J Public Health 91:1056–1059, 2001.
65. Gillespie LD, Gillespie WJ, Cumming R, et al: Interventions to reduce the incidence of falling in the elderly. Cochrane Database Syst Rev, 1999.
66. Whipple RH, Wolfson LI, Amerman PM: The relationship of knee and ankle to falls in nursing home residents: An isokinetic study. J Am Geriatr Soc 35:13–20, 1987.
67. Allen SH: Exercise considerations for postmenopausal women with osteoporosis. Arthritis Care Res 7:205–214, 1994.
68. Honkanen R, Tuppurainen M, Kroger H, et al: Relationships between risk factors and fractures differ by type of fracture: a population-based study of 12,192 perimenopausal women. Osteoporos Int 8:25–31, 1998.
69. Siris ES, Miller PD, Barrett-Connor E, et al: Identification and fracture outcomes of undiagnosed low bone mineral density in postmenopausal women: results from the National Osteoporosis Risk Assessment. JAMA 286:2815–2822, 2001.
70. Tuppurainen M, Kroger H, Honkanen R, et al: Risks of perimenopausal fractures: a prospective population-based study. Acta Obstet Gynecol Scand 74:624–628, 1995.
71. Fujiwara S, Kasagi F, Yamada M, et al: Risk factors for hip fracture in a Japanese cohort. J Bone Miner Res 12:998–1004, 1997.
72. Kelepouris N, Harper KD, Gannon F, et al: Severe osteoporosis in men. Ann Intern Med 123:452–460, 1995.
73. Tinetti ME, Speechley M, Ginter SF: Risk factors for falls among elderly persons living in the community. N Engl J Med 319:1701–1707, 1998.
74. Grisso JA, Kelsey JL, Strom BL, et al, and the Northeast Hip Fracture Study Group: Risk factors for falls as a cause of hip fracture in women. N Engl J Med 324:1326–1331, 1991.
75. Tinetti ME, Baker DI, McAvay G, et al: A multifactorial intervention to reduce the risk of falling among elderly people living in the community. J Engl J Med 331:821–827, 1994.
76. Gill TM, Baker DI, Gottschalk M, et al: A program to prevent functional decline in physically frail, elderly persons who live at home. N Engl J Med 347:1068–1074, 2002.
77. Jensen J, Lundin-Olsson L, Nyberg L, et al: Fall and injury prevention in older people living in residential care facilities. Ann Intern Med 136:733–741, 2002.
78. Kannus P, Parkkari J, Niemi S, et al: Prevention of hip fracture in elderly people with use of a hip protector. N Engl J Med 343; 1506–1513, 2000.

Treatment of Osteoporosis: Pharmacologic

chapter 7

Michael T. McDermott, M.D.,
Carol Zapalowski, M.D., Ph.D.,
and Paul D. Miller, M.D.

The goal of osteoporosis treatment is to prevent fragility fractures. Interventions should be demonstrated to reduce fractures effectively and safely. The highest level of evidence for efficacy and safety is the randomized controlled trial (RCT). In the discussion that follows, we will outline the currently used strategies for osteoporosis management, citing, whenever possible, data from RCTs that used fracture reduction as their primary endpoint.

Bone Remodeling

Bone remodeling is the process by which older, weaker bone tissue is removed and replaced by newer, stronger bone tissue. This process is a continuous one that is ongoing simultaneously at millions of sites throughout the entire skeleton. Bone remodeling consists of three main processes: bone resorption, bone formation, and bone mineralization (Fig. 7-1). Osteoclasts are multinucleated giant cells that develop from hematopoietic stem cell precursors. Activated osteoclasts bind along their ruffled borders to internal bone surfaces and secrete acid, proteolytic enzymes, and free radicals, which dissolve the underlying bone, leaving resorption pits. As osteoclasts migrate along bone surfaces, they also release cytokines that activate nearby osteoblasts, which develop from mesenchymal cell precursors. Multiple osteoblasts are recruited into recently excavated resorption pits and refill these cavities by secreting osteoid, a bone-specific collagen. If the calcium and phosphate concentrations in the circulation and extracelluar fluid are adequate, calcium-phosphate (hydroxyapatite) crystals precipitate into the new osteoid, causing it to harden and mature. Osteocytes then develop from mature osteoblasts and reside in crevices within bone tissue. These cells act as mechanoreceptors that sense developing areas of skeletal stress

71

Figure 7-1. Bone remodeling is a continual process throughout the skeleton. Osteoclastic bone (OC) resorption removes old bone, leaving resorption pits. Osteoblasts (OB) then secrete osteoid into the newly excavated spaces. Mineralization follows as calcium phosphate (hydroxyapatite) crystals precipitate in the newly laid osteoid to solidify and stabilize the newly formed bone tissue.

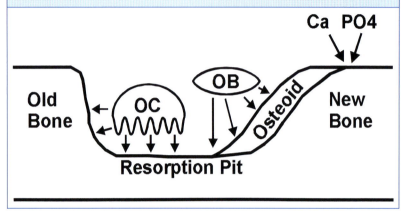

and then orchestrate local bone remodeling by sending signals to the other bone cells to activate or suppress new bone remodeling units in the appropriate areas.

Strategies of Pharmacologic Intervention in Osteoporosis

Pharmacologic treatment of osteoporosis entails administering medications that favorably alter bone remodeling. Current strategies include agents that inhibit osteoclastic bone resorption (antiresorptive agents) and agents that stimulate osteoblastic bone formation (anabolic agents; see Table 7-1). Antiresorptive agents increase bone mass by inhibiting bone resorption without initially affecting bone formation. Consequently, in the first 1–2 years of their use, bone formation exceeds bone resorption,

Table 7-1.	Current Treatment Strategies	
	Agent	**Action**
Antiresorptive	Bisphosphonates Raloxifene Calcitonin Estrogen	Inhibit osteoclastic bone resorption
Anabolic	Parathyroid hormone	Stimulate osteoblastic bone formation

Figure 7-2. BMD increases during osteoporosis therapy. The mechanisms underlying these BMD increments and the patterns of change over time differ with the two categories of medications. *Antiresorptive agents* rapidly inhibit bone resorption without affecting bone formation, resulting in a period (12–18 months) during which bone formation exceeds resorption, and significant increases in BMD occur. Bone formation eventually drops, however, because of resorption-formation coupling mechanisms, and BMD stabilizes or increases only modestly thereafter. *Anabolic agents* stimulate new bone formation, producing progressive increments in BMD and new trabecular bone elements. Whether compensatory increases in bone resorption will subsequently limit the degree of BMD gain with more prolonged use has yet to be determined.

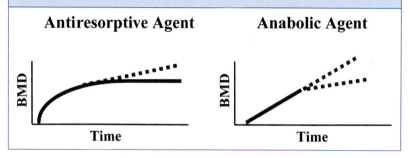

producing a net increase in bone mass. This is known as the bone remodeling transient. Because bone cells signal to one another to maintain appropriate resorption-formation coupling, the rate of bone formation eventually decreases to equal that of resorption, and bone mass tends to stabilize with only modest or no additional major gains thereafter (Fig. 7-2). Anabolic agents, in contrast, increase bone mass by stimulating new bone formation; longer studies will be necessary to determine whether they will produce continuous linear increments or whether subsequent increases in bone resorption will limit the magnitude of the bone mass gains achieved. The mechanisms by which antiresorptive medications reduce fractures relate both to the rapid decrease in bone resorption and microporosity and to the more gradual increase in bone mass that occurs during the first 1–2 years of their use (Fig. 7-3). For anabolic agents, fracture reduction seems to be due primarily to the resulting progressive bone mass increments and the formation of new trabecular bone elements.

The National Osteoporosis Foundation (Table 7-2) recommends initiating therapy in all patients who have T scores < –2.0, if they have no other risk factors, and in those who have T scores < –1.5, if at least one other risk factor is present.

Figure 7-3. Fracture risk decreases with osteoporosis therapy. The mechanisms underlying this effect differ with the two types of medication. *Antiresorptive agents* reduce fracture risk initially by rapidly decreasing bone resorption and bone microporosity and by subsequent increases in BMD. *Anabolic agents* reduce fracture risk by progressively increasing BMD, increasing the number of bony trabeculae in cancellous bone, and increasing bone size.

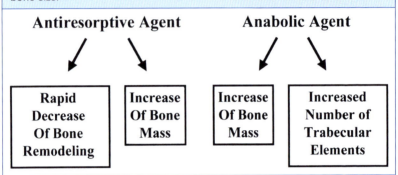

Table 7-2.	Patient Selection for Treatment with Pharmacologic Therapy

A. All patients who have had a fragility fracture
B. Patients with a T score < –2.0 on central bone densitometry
C. Patients with a T score < –1.5 on central bone densitometry, if they have one or more additional risk factors for fractures

From Pocket Guide to Prevention and Treatment of Osteoporosis. National Osteoporosis Foundation, 1998. www.nof.org.

Antiresorptive Therapy

Bisphosphonates

The bisphosphonates are a group of agents that avidly bind to hydroxyapatite crystals in bone. When activated osteoclasts attempt to resorb bone to which bisphosphonates are bound, these medications inhibit osteoclast function and promote osteoclast cell death (apoptosis). Although many bisphosphonates are available or are in development, at the time of this writing only two, alendronate (Fosamax) and risedronate (Actonel) are approved by the FDA for use in the prevention and treatment of osteoporosis. They are the only medications for which there is published evidence documenting efficacy in the reduction of both vertebral and hip fractures. Oral ibandronate (Boniva) is also FDA approved but not yet available.

Alendronate was shown in the FIT 1 trial[1] to significantly reduce bone resorption biomarkers by 59% (vs. placebo) and to increase BMD by 6.2% (vs. placebo) in the lumbar spine and by 4.1% (vs. placebo) in the femoral neck when given for 3 years to women with post-menopausal osteoporosis and previous vertebral fractures. More importantly, it was shown to reduce the relative risk of new vertebral fractures by 47% (P <0.001 vs. placebo) and the relative risk of hip fractures by 51% (P = 0.04 vs. placebo). An open-label extension of the FIT 1 trial reported that patients maintained on the 10-mg daily oral dose for a period of 7–10 years had a continuous increase in spine BMD of 0.7% per year after the first 18 months, resulting in an overall 10-year mean increment of 13%; hip BMD remained stable throughout this same period after the initial increment in the first 18 months of treatment.[2,3] A large meta-analysis[4] of alendronate treatment RCTs that had been completed by 2002 reported that alendronate increased lumbar spine BMD by an average of 7.36% and reduced the risk of vertebral fractures by 47% (RR, 0.53; 95% CI, 0.43–0.65) and of nonvertebral fractures by 51% (RR, 0.49; 95% CI, 0.36–0.67). A 70-mg weekly dose of alen-dronate has been shown to increase spine and hip BMD to the same degree as the 10-mg daily dose[5]; however, fracture reduction efficacy has not yet been reported with weekly dosing.

Risedronate was shown in the VERT NA study[6] to decrease bone resorption biomarkers by 30% (vs. placebo) and to increase BMD by 4.3% (vs. placebo) in the lumbar spine and by 2.8% (vs. placebo) in the femoral neck over the 3-year study duration in women with post-menopausal osteoporosis and previous vertebral fractures. The relative risk of new vertebral fractures was reduced by 65% after just 1 year (P < 0.001 vs. placebo) and by 41% after 3 years (P = 0.003 vs. placebo) of treatment. The VERT MN study,[7] a concurrent RCT conducted in Europe, showed similar reductions in new vertebral fractures of 61% after 1 year (P < 0.001 vs. placebo) and 49% after 3 years (P < 0.001 vs. placebo). A 2-year extension of VERT MN,[8] that maintained the ran-domized controlled design, reported persistent benefits, with an overall 9.3% increase in spine BMD (P < 0.01 vs. placebo) and an additional 59% reduction during year 4-5 in new vertebral fractures (P < 0.01 vs. placebo) over the 5-year study duration. The HIP trial,[9] the only study to use hip fractures as a primary end point, examined the effects of ris-edronate in 70- to 79-year-old women with documented osteoporosis (low BMD group) and in women ≥ 80 years old with clinical risk factors but no BMD requirement for entry (clinical risk factor group). The rela-tive risk reduction for hip fractures was 30% for the entire group (P = 0.02 vs. placebo), 40% for the 70- to 79-year-old low-BMD group (P < 0.009 vs. placebo), and 60% for women who had experienced previous vertebral fractures. A 2002 meta-analysis[4] of risedronate treatment RCTs reported that risedronate increased lumbar spine BMD by an average of

4.53% and reduced the risk of vertebral fractures by 36% (RR, 0.64; 95% CI, 0.54–0.77) and of nonvertebral fractures by 27% (RR, 0.73; 95% CI, 0.61–0.87). A 35-mg weekly dose of risedronate has also been reported to produce spine and hip BMD increments that are similar to those seen with the 5-mg daily dose[10]; however, fracture reduction data for the weekly dose are not yet available.

Alendronate (Fosamax) is available in 10-mg tablets for daily use and 70-mg tablets for weekly use. Risedronate (Actonel) is available in 5-mg tablets and 35-mg tablets for daily and weekly use, respectively. The only major side effect with these agents has been gastroesophageal irritation, which causes symptoms in approximately 1% of treated patients (compared with placebo). This side effect can be decreased or eliminated in most patients by emphasizing the proper method of use. Both agents are best taken in the morning on an empty stomach with a full 8 oz. of water. Patients should then remain upright and should ingest no food and take no medications, vitamins, or calcium supplements for at least 30 minutes afterwards. These measures help to minimize the possibility of esophageal irritation and to maximize intestinal absorption of the medication.

Other bisphosphonates are currently available or are under investigation but, at present, are either not FDA approved for the prevention or treatment of osteoporosis or are not yet available. These include etidronate (Didronel), pamidronate (Aredia), zoledronic acid (Zometa), and ibandronate (Boniva). Etidronate, given orally as 200 mg twice a day for 2 weeks followed by 2½ months of calcium and vitamin D supplements in repeated cycles, was reported to increase lumbar spine BMD by 2.8%–8.0% (vs. placebo) and to reduce the relative risk of new vertebral fractures by at least 50% after 2 years of use.[11,12] However, questionable long-term (3 years) antifracture efficacy has prevented its approval by the FDA. Pamidronate, given as 30 mg intravenously every 3 months for a period of 2 years, has been reported[13] to increase spine BMD by 10% (vs. baseline) and femoral neck BMD by 4.8% (vs. baseline). Intravenous zoledronic acid has been shown to increase spine BMD by 4.3%–5.1% (vs. placebo) and femoral neck BMD by 3.1%–3.5% (vs. placebo) after 1 year regardless of whether it was given as 0.25–1.0 mg every 3 months, 2 mg every 6 months, or 4 mg as a single dose.[14] Intravenous ibandronate, given in doses ranging from 0.5–2.0 mg every 3 months, has been reported to increase BMD in the spine by 2.7%–4.4% (vs. placebo) and by 1.8%–2.9% (vs. placebo) in the total hip, but it did not significantly alter BMD in the femoral neck.[15] At present, there are no fracture reduction data for any of these three intravenous bisphosphonates. Convincing antifracture efficacy and safety data will be necessary for FDA approval.

When a provider determines that a bisphosphonate is the appropriate agent for a patient, we recommend that one of the two FDA-approved oral bisphosphonates (alendronate, risedronate) be pre-scribed. Etidronate can be used as an alternative when cost is a major issue or in some cases when there are side effects from alendronate and risedronate. An intravenous bisphosphonate (pamidronate, zoledronic acid) can be considered in patients who are unable to tolerate or who seem not to be adequately absorbing an oral bisphosphonate.

Raloxifene

Raloxifene (Evista) belongs to a class of drugs known as selective estrogen receptor modulators (SERMs). These medications bind to estro-gen receptors but selectively function as estrogen agonists in some tis-sues and as estrogen antagonists in other tissues. Raloxifene is an estrogen agonist in bone and an estrogen antagonist in the breast and uterus. Raloxifene is currently FDA approved for both the prevention and treatment of postmenopausal osteoporosis (Table 7-3). No other SERM has yet been approved for this condition.

Raloxifene was shown in the MORE trial[16] to reduce bone resorption biomarkers by 26% (vs. placebo), to increase spine BMD by 2.6% (vs. placebo), and to increase femoral neck BMD by 2.1% (vs. placebo). After 2–3 years of treatment, the risk of new vertebral fractures was reduced by 50% in women who had no preexisting vertebral fractures ($P < 0.05$ vs. placebo) and by 30% in women with previous vertebral fractures ($P < 0.05$ vs. placebo). A subsequent post hoc analysis of this trial reported that new clinical (symptomatic) vertebral fractures were reduced by 68% (RR, 0.32; 95% CI, 0.13–0.80) in the first year of ralox-ifene therapy.[17] An extension of the study for an additional year showed persistence of effect, with a 4-year vertebral fracture risk reduction of 49% (RR, 0.51; 95% CI, 0.35–0.73) in women without prevalent verte-bral fractures and 34% (RR, 0.66; 95% CI, 0.55–0.81) in women with prevalent vertebral fractures.[18] In the MORE study, there was also

Table 7-3.	Medications that are Currently FDA Approved for the Prevention and Treatment of Osteoporosis	
	FDA Approval	
	Prevention	*Treatment*
Antiresorptive Agents		
Alendronate	Yes	Yes
Risedronate	Yes	Yes
Raloxifene	Yes	Yes
Calcitonin	No	Yes
Estrogen	Yes	No
Anabolic Agents		
Teriparatide	No	Yes

evidence that raloxifene might decrease the risk of breast cancer[19] and the risk of cardiovascular disease in high-risk postmenopausal women.[20] Further studies to confirm these preliminary findings are ongoing, because these were not primary end points of the MORE trial.

Raloxifene is available in 60-mg tablets, which are recommended for osteoporosis prevention and treatment. The most prominent side effects include hot flashes in some individuals and an increased risk of venous thrombosis (blood clots) developing.

Calcitonin

Calcitonin is a hormone that is naturally produced by the parafollicular C cells of the thyroid gland. Its primary function is to inhibit osteoclastic bone resorption. Human calcitonin is a relatively weak hormone, whereas salmon make a more potent species. Synthetic salmon calcitonin has therefore been developed as a treatment option for patients with osteoporosis. Calcitonin (Miacalcin) is currently FDA approved for the treatment but not for the prevention of postmenopausal osteoporosis.

In the PROOF study,[21] intranasal calcitonin increased spine BMD by 0.7%, and the 200 IU daily dose (but not the 100 IU or the 400 IU daily doses) reduced the relative risk of new vertebral fractures by 33% ($P = 0.03$ vs. placebo). A 2002 meta-analysis[4] of all calcitonin treatment RCTs reported that calcitonin increased BMD in the lumbar spine by an average of 3.7% and that it reduced the risk of vertebral fractures by 54% (RR, 0.46; 95% CI, 0.25–0.87) and of nonvertebral fractures by a statistically nonsignificant 48% (RR, 0.52; 95% CI, 0.22–1.23). No studies were adequately powered to evaluate the antifracture efficacy of calcitonin in the hip. Calcitonin given intranasally or subcutaneously has also been reported to have mild to moderate analgesic effects in some patients and may therefore have a role in the treatment of patients with back pain resulting from recent vertebral fractures. Calcitonin is available as intranasal and subcutaneous preparations. The main side effects are occasional nasal irritation (rhinitis).

Estrogen

Estrogen has long been known to have beneficial skeletal effects in postmenopausal women. At present, estrogen replacement is FDA approved for the prevention but not for the treatment of postmenopausal osteoporosis. Tremendous controversy exists, however, regarding the overall risk/benefit profile of taking this hormone.

The Women's Health Initiative (WHI; described later) 5.2-year interim analysis[22] of their Premarin plus Provera group (HRT group) reported that combined hormone replacement reduced the risk of new vertebral fractures by 34% (RR, 0.66; 95% CI, 0.44–0.98) and the risk of hip fractures also by 34% (RR, 0.66; 95% CI, 0.45–0.98). Data on women taking estrogen alone because of a prior hysterectomy will not be available until the full trial is complete in 2004. The 2002 meta-analysis[4] of all available estrogen treatment trials, excluding the WHI study, reported that estrogens produce a mean increment in spine BMD of 6.8% after 2 years of treatment but statistically nonsignificant risk reductions of 34% for vertebral fractures (RR, 0.66; 95% CI, 0.41–1.07) and of 13% for nonvertebral fractures (RR, 0.87; 95% CI, 0.71–1.08).

Estrogens may be administered as oral conjugated estrogens (Premarin, Cenestin), esterified estrogens (Estratabs, Menest), estropipate (Ogen, Ortho-Est, Estropipate), estradiol (Estrace, Gynodiol, Estradiol), ethinyl estradiol (Estinyl), or transdermal estradiol patches (Estraderm, Vivelle, Climara, Alora, Esclim, FemPatch). Oral progestins that are commonly used include medroxyprogesterone acetate (Provera, Cycrin, Amen, Curretab, Medroxyprogesterone), norethindrone acetate (Aygestin), and micronized progesterone (Prometrium). Combined estrogen/progestin products include oral conjugated estrogens plus medroxyprogesterone (PremPro, PremPhase), estradiol plus norethindrone (Activella), ethinyl estradiol plus norethindrone (FemHRT), estradiol plus norgestimate (Ortho-Prefest), and transdermal estradiol plus norethindrone patches (Combipatch). Combined oral esterified estrogen plus methyltestosterone (Estratest, Estratest HS) is also available.

The controversy surrounding the use of hormone replacement therapy (HRT) has been fueled by several recent publications. The HERS study[23] prospectively examined use of combined Premarin/Provera compared with placebo in 2763 postmenopausal women (mean age, 67 years) with known coronary artery disease (CAD). In the first year after initiation of HRT, there was a significant 52% increase of CAD events (hazard ratio, 1.52; 95% CI, 1.01–2.29); this increased risk was present only during the first year and did not persist in the subsequent 4 years of the study. However, the anticipated reduction in CAD risk was clearly not seen with HRT. The HERS II extension study[24,25] confirmed the lack of CAD protection with more prolonged HRT use in this population and reported a statistically significant doubling of the risk of deep vein thrombosis developing ($P < 0.02$).

The WHI[22] is an ongoing large prospective study designed to evaluate the effects of multiple interventions (nutrition modification, calcium and vitamin D supplementation, HRT) on the risks for CAD, invasive breast cancer, colon cancer, and skeletal fractures in 161,809 postmenopausal women. The hormone replacement segment of this study enrolled 27,347 women (age range, 50–79 years; mean age, 63 years) and had a planned duration of 8 years with interim analyses for safety.

The 10,739 women who had previously undergone hysterectomies were randomly assigned to receive either conjugated estrogens (ERT group) or placebo. The 16,608 women who had not had hysterectomies were randomly assigned to receive either conjugated estrogens plus medroxyprogesterone (HRT group) or placebo. At the 5.2-year interim analysis, the adverse event data was sufficiently compelling to cause the investigators to terminate the HRT arm and to publish the results.[22,26–28] The ERT arm was terminated in 2004, and the data are being prepared for publication.

The findings from the prematurely terminated HRT arm of the WHI were that HRT was associated with a 29% increased risk of coronary heart disease (hazard ratio, 1.29; nominal 95% CI, 1.02–1.63), a 26% increased risk of invasive breast cancer (hazard ratio, 1.26; nominal 95% CI, 1.00–1.59), a 41% increased risk of stroke (hazard ratio, 1.41; nominal 95% CI, 1.07–1.85), and a 110% increased risk of venous thromboembolism (hazard ratio, 2.11; nominal 95% CI, 1.58–2.82). Conversely, the risk of colon cancer was reduced by 37% (hazard ratio, 0.63; nominal 95% CI, 0.43–0.92), and, as discussed previously, the risk of vertebral or hip fractures was each reduced by 34%. Attributable risk analysis determined that if 2000 postmenopausal women were given HRT for 5 years (10,000 patient-years), there would be seven excess cases of coronary heart disease, eight additional cases of invasive breast cancer, eight more strokes, and eight more thromboembolic events, whereas there would be six fewer cases of colon cancer and five fewer hip fractures. A subsequent report from the HRT portion of the WHI disappointingly showed that combined estrogen and progesterone therapy had no significant effect on quality-of-life measures other than vasomotor symptoms in women age 50–54 years.[26] Additional WHI reports, evaluating a subset of women who were 65 years of age or older, indicated that HRT had no significant benefit on cognitive function[27] and seemed to actually double the risk of probable dementia developing (hazard ratio, 2.05; 95% CI, 1.21–3.48).[28]

The American College of Obstetrics and Gynecology (ACOG) issued a statement in response to the findings of the WHI HRT arm. They recommended that each woman discuss these matters with her primary care provider and/or gynecologist to determine what the risks and benefits of short-term or long-term HRT use would be for her individually. We agree with this position. We recommend, however, that women whose HRT is discontinued be considered for bone densitometry testing and fracture risk assessment in order to determine whether other interventions for the prevention or treatment of osteoporosis should be instituted.

Phytoestrogens are plant molecules that have estrogen-like activity. Isoflavones, the phytoestrogens found in abundance in soybeans and soy-derived products, are the most widely studied. The most efficacious isoflavones are genistein and diadzen. A study comparing genistein to HRT[29] in early postmenopausal women (age 47–57 years old) reported that genistein reduced bone resorption biomarkers by 43% ($P < 0.001$ vs. placebo; P = ns vs. HRT) and increased formation biomarkers by 23%–29% ($P < 0.03$ vs. placebo), whereas HRT was found to reduce formation markers by 17%–20%. Genistein increased spine BMD 4.6% ($P < 0.001$ vs. placebo) and femoral neck BMD 4.25% ($P < 0.001$ vs. placebo); these BMD increments were comparable to those seen with HRT (P = ns). Further studies will be necessary to demonstrate whether or not these agents have antifracture efficacy and to determine long-term safety. Once these issues are resolved, however, phytoestrogens may be a novel approach to the prevention and treatment of post-menopausal osteoporosis.

Anabolic Therapy

Until the release of injectable human parathyroid hormone (recombinant human PTH [1-34]), all of the FDA-approved medications to prevent and treat osteoporosis were antiresorptive agents, which inhibit osteoclastic bone resorption. This action allows bone formation to transiently exceed bone resorption, resulting in a modest increase in bone mass and a reduced fracture risk. Anabolic agents, on the other hand, stimulate bone formation through direct effects on the osteoblasts and marrow stromal cells. The osteoblasts release local cytokines, which lead to a parallel increase in osteoclast activity. This class of drugs therefore activates the entire bone remodeling cycle. The relatively greater increase in osteoblastic activity allows the formation of new bone and a subsequent increase in bone density. When used in the proper doses, this translates into an increase in bone strength and decrease in fracture risk.

Serum and urinary biochemical markers of bone turnover are often used to assess effects of various medications and disease states on bone. Bone markers are used to help determine whether medications are having an effect on bone formation, bone resorption, or both. Most of these markers are clinically available in commercial laboratories. Markers of bone formation include bone-specific alkaline phosphatase, osteocalcin, and C-terminal propeptide of type 1 procollagen (P1CP) or N-terminal propeptide (P1NP). Markers of bone resorption include N-telopeptide (NTx), C-telopeptide (CTx), and deoxypyridinoline (DpD).

The compounds that are considered anabolic to the skeleton include fluoride, strontium, anabolic steroids, growth hormone (GH), insulin-like growth factor-1 (IGF-1), statins, and PTH. None but rhPTH (1-34) has been FDA approved for the indication of osteoporosis.

Parathyroid Hormone

PTH and 1,25 dihydroxyvitamin D_3 are the primary regulators of calcium homeostasis (Fig. 7-4). In bone, PTH is involved in the release of calcium and phosphate. In the kidney, it stimulates reabsorption of calcium and inhibits the reabsorption of phosphate. PTH also stimulates renal 1α-hydroxylase activity, leading to an increase in the synthesis of 1,25 dihydroxyvitamin D_3, the biologically active form of vitamin D. 1,25 Dihydroxyvitamin D_3 increases the intestinal absorption of calcium

Figure 7-4. PTH and 1,25 dihydroxyvitamin D regulate calcium homeostasis. PTH secreted from the parathyroid glands increases the serum calcium concentration by stimulating osteoclastic bone resorption, renal tubular calcium reabsorption, and renal 1 alpha-hydroxylase activity, which converts circulating 25 hydroxyvitamin D to 1,25 dihydroxyvitamin D. The latter also increases the serum calcium level by stimulating intestinal calcium absorption and bone resorption.

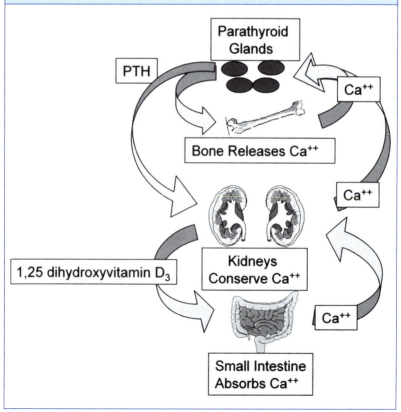

and phosphate. Extracellular calcium is the most important regulator of PTH secretion.[30,31]

PTH is secreted as a single-chain polypeptide, consisting of 84 amino acids (PTH 1-84). The amino terminal region of PTH is the most biologically active, and in fact, PTH (1-34) (Fig. 7-5) has nearly the same biologic activity as the full 84 amino acid molecule, PTH (1-84).

Fuller Albright and Hans Selye[32,33] were the first to show that parathyroid extract could increase bone mass in rodents. PTH was synthesized, and human trials began in the 1970s. Intermittent, subcutaneous injections of PTH in humans have been shown to increase BMD at the spine and the hip,[34–36] and to reduce the risk of vertebral and nonvertebral fractures.[34] The majority of trials have used human PTH (hPTH) (1-34), and therefore conclusions about any relative advantages of hPTH (1-34) or hPTH (1-84) are not possible.

Recombinant hPTH (1-34) has been FDA approved for treatment of severe osteoporosis. This compound is also known as teriparatide, hPTH (1-34), rhPTH (1-34), and Forteo.

It is interesting to think of PTH as an anabolic agent. In hyperparathyroidism, during which there is continuous excess secretion of PTH, a catabolic response on the skeleton is seen. The increase in

Figure 7-5. Human parathyroid hormone. The intact PTH molecule is 84 amino acids long. Teriparatide is recombinant human PTH truncated to the first 34 amino acids. Teriparatide is FDA approved for treatment of osteoporosis in the dose of 20 μg given subcutaneously daily.

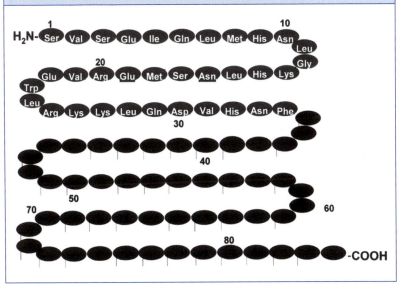

osteoclast activity and increased bone resorption results in a loss of bone mass. The response is quite different when PTH is administered subcutaneously in a low-dose, intermittent fashion. The predominant effect with a daily low-dose injection of PTH is on the osteoblast rather than on the osteoclast. With intermittent administration of PTH, there is decreased osteoblast apoptosis, increased osteoblast number and function, and increased bone formation, and therefore increased bone mass and bone strength (Fig. 7-6). Administration of intermittent PTH has been shown to increase trabecular bone volume, trabecular connectivity, bone size, and strength.

Treatment with rhPTH (1-34) results, initially, in an increase in the bone formation markers, bone-specific alkaline phosphatase, and osteocalcin. This is followed by a slower increase in bone resorption, as evidenced by an increase in urinary N-telopeptide excretion.[37,38] This suggests an earlier effect on bone formation, followed by a subsequent increase in overall bone turnover.

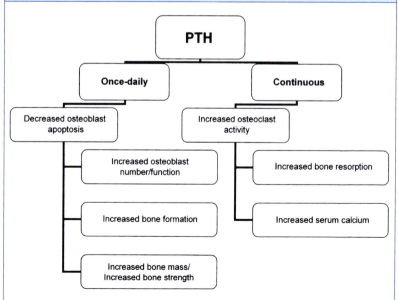

Figure 7-6. Variable effects of PTH depending on dosing regimen. The skeletal effects of PTH depend on the pattern of the dosing regimen or systemic exposure. PTH given once daily preferentially stimulates osteoblast activity over osteoclast activity, resulting in stimulation of new bone formation. Continuous exposure to PTH, either exogenous or endogenous, preferentially stimulates bone resorption more than bone formation.

When PTH was first evaluated for clinical use, there was concern about the potential loss of cortical bone. This concern arose for several reasons. It is known that there is preferential cortical bone loss in patients with primary hyperparathyroidism. In studies with PTH (1-34), bone density at the one-third wrist, an area of highly cortical bone, either remained stable or decreased. However, PTH has also been shown to increase periosteal bone formation, periosteal circumference, and cortical thickness in human bone. All these are predictive of increased biomechanical strength. Furthermore, Neer et al[34], showed a reduction in fractures of the nonvertebral skeleton, which would be unlikely if PTH was negatively affecting cortical bone.

Neer et al[34] conducted an RCT with 1637 postmenopausal women, all of whom had prior vertebral fractures. The women received either placebo, 20 µg of hPTH (1-34) or 40 µg of hPTH (1-34), given as a daily subcutaneous injection for a median treatment period of 21 months. The average age of these women was 69 years, and, at baseline, they had an average of two to three vertebral fractures. Compared with placebo, 20 µg and 40-µg doses of hPTH (1-34) increased BMD at the lumbar spine by 9% and 13%, respectively; BMD was increased by 3% and 6%, respectively, at the femoral neck and by 2.6% and 3.6%, respectively, at the total hip. PTH, at the 20-µg/day and 40-µg/day dose, reduced the risk of one or more new vertebral fractures by 65% and 69%, respectively (Fig. 7-7). Nonvertebral fractures were reduced by 53% and 54%, respectively (Fig. 7-8). The trial was not statistically powered to show a significant decrease in hip fracture.

The major side effects were nausea, headache, and leg cramps. Side effects were significantly more frequent in the 40-µg group. In addition, sustained increases in calcium above the normal range occurred in 3% of the 20-µg group and 11% of the 40-µg group. Urinary calcium increased by 30 mg per 24 hours in the treatment groups, on average. There was no increase in the incidence of hypercalciuria or renal calculi in either group.

Orwoll et al[38] looked at the effects of teriparatide hPTH (1-34) on bone density in osteoporotic men. 437 men with either idiopathic osteoporosis or osteoporosis associated with hypogonadism were randomly assigned to placebo or teriparatide. The trial was stopped at 11 months, at which time BMD in the lumbar spine had increased by 6% and 9% in the 20-µg and 40-µg groups, respectively. Femoral neck BMD increased 1.5% and 2.9% in the two treatment groups, respectively. There was no change in radial bone density with teriparatide administration. This increase was irrespective of gonadal status. The trial was stopped at 11 months because of the finding of an increased incidence of osteosarcoma in rats, discussed later.

Figure 7-7. Effect of PTH on the risk of new vertebral fractures. This randomized controlled trial included 1637 postmenopausal women with prior vertebral fractures. They were randomly assigned to either 20 μg or 40 μg of recombinant human PTH or placebo given as a subcutaneous injection daily. The median treatment time was 19 months, and the women, on average, were 69 years old, with an average of two to three vertebral fractures at baseline. There was a statistically significant decrease in the number of new vertebral fractures: 65% in women who used the 20-μg dose and 69% in women using the 40-μg dose. (Adapted from Neer RM, Arnaud CD, Zanchetta JR, et al: Effect of parathyroid hormone (1–34) on fractures and bone mineral density in postmenopausal women with osteoporosis. N Engl J Med 344:1434–1441, 2001.)

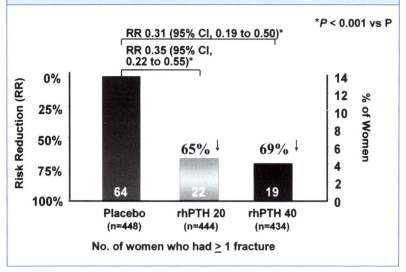

Kurland et al[39] studied 23 men with idiopathic osteoporosis treated with daily subcutaneous injections of human PTH 1-34 at a dose equivalent to 25-μg for 18 months and showed a BMD increase at the lumbar spine of 13.5% compared with placebo.

In a safety study in rats, hPTH (1-34) was administered for 18–24 months, starting with 6-week-old rats.[40] In these animals, there was a significant increase in the incidence of osteogenic sarcoma that was dose dependent and related to duration of use. Giving PTH for this duration of time and starting at this early age is essentially equivalent to a lifetime exposure to an agent that increases osteoblast proliferation. However, there has been no increase in osteosarcoma in primate studies of PTH administration, and there has been only one case thus far in the literature of osteogenic sarcoma developing in a patient with hyperparathyroidism. None of the 1637 patients in the Neer trial[34] have developed osteogenic sarcoma develop. And finally, osteogenic sarcoma has

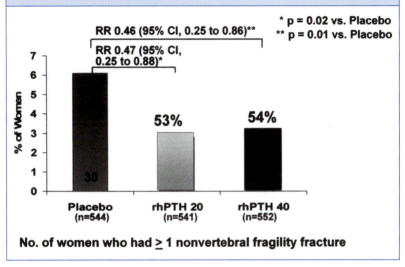

Figure 7-8. Effect of PTH on the risk of nonvertebral fragility fractures. This randomized controlled trial included 1637 postmenopausal women with prior vertebral fractures. They were randomly assigned to either 20 μg or 40 μg of recombinant human PTH or placebo given as a subcutaneous injection daily. The median treatment time was 19 months, and the women, on average, were 69 years old, with an average of two to three vertebral fractures at baseline. There was a statistically significant decrease in the risk for nonvertebral fragility fractures in both tested doses. (Adapted from Neer RM, Arnaud CD, Zanchetta JR, et al: Effect of parathyroid hormone (1–34) on fractures and bone mineral density in postmenopausal women with osteoporosis. N Engl J Med 344:1434–1441, 2001.)

not been associated with parathyroid cancer, a disease in which PTH levels are very high, nor end-stage renal disease, which has the highest PTH levels of any chronic disease state.

For the reasons just discussed, it is reasonable to assume that PTH is safe when administered to humans, although continued postmarketing surveillance and further safety data are needed. There are groups for whom PTH is not recommended because of a known or theoretical increased risk for osteosarcoma. These include patients with Paget's disease, who are known to have a slightly increased risk of sarcoma. In addition, anyone with any unexplained increase in alkaline phosphatase, anyone ever diagnosed with a primary bone cancer or a cancer metastatic to bone, anyone having had radiation therapy to bone, and anyone with hypercalciuria or an elevated PTH level should not be treated with PTH. In addition, it is not recommended that PTH be used in growing children or young adults. The *Physicians' Desk Reference* has a black box warning for recombinant hPTH (1-34) (teriparatide [Forteo]), which describes the increased incidence of osteosarcoma reported in these rat studies.

PTH is therefore a very promising new medication and the only FDA-approved anabolic agent for osteoporosis. It has been shown to produce impressive increases in BMD and to decrease the risk for both vertebral and nonverterbral fractures. To date, no significant reduction of hip fracture has been demonstrated. More studies are required to determine long-term safety and the effect of PTH on hip fracture reduction.

Fluoride

Sodium fluoride was the first anabolic agent to be used in the treatment of postmenopausal osteoporosis. Fluoride is an essential trace element. Like other trace elements, adequate intake of fluoride is essential for normal growth and development, but pharmacologic doses can be toxic.[41] Fluoride treatment results in a dramatic increase in BMD in patients with osteoporosis. Increases in the number of osteoblasts and the number of osteoblast-covered surfaces suggest that the rise in bone mass seen with fluoride therapy is due to an increase in osteoblast function. The earliest studies with fluoride were done with high doses (75 mg/day), which produced marked increases in BMD at the spine. Despite these significant increases, however, there was no reduction in vertebral fractures and a possible increase in nonvertebral fractures. In addition, fluoride caused significant gastrointestinal side effects and a lower extremity pain syndrome.[41–43]

Fluoride was subsequently studied with lower dose, slow-release formulations.[44] The increases in bone mass were not as significant as those seen with the higher doses, but there were significant reductions in vertebral fractures, and the incidence of adverse side effects was significantly less.

Fluoride has a very narrow therapeutic window. This element can accumulate in bone, replacing calcium in hydroxyapatite, and may thereby cause harmful effects on bone quality and strength. It is not known at what point the accumulation of fluoride in the skeleton starts to have a negative effect on bone quality. When the toxic threshold for skeletal fluoride is exceeded, bone shows evidence of sclerosis. This includes abnormal bone formation, impaired mineralization, and reduced bone strength.

Fluoride administration can result in osteomalacia, a disorder of mineralization of newly formed bone matrix that occurs in adults. In a study by Riggs et al,[42] osteomalacia was seen in transiliac crest biopsies, despite the fact that the patients had been supplemented with 1500 mg of calcium per day. It is possible that adequate supplementation with calcium and vitamin D may be able to prevent this effect, but the doses of calcium and vitamin D necessary to prevent osteomalacia are unknown.

Treatment with fluoride results in an increase in the bone formation markers, bone-specific alkaline phosphatase, and osteocalcin. Because fluoride therapy can lead to osteomalacia, which is also associated with an increase in these biomarkers, it is not clear that an increase in these biomarkers with fluoride therapy is advantageous to bone.[41]

Fluoride, therefore, has the potential to be an efficacious agent in osteoporosis. When administered in low dosage, it also has the advantage of being less expensive than some of the other anabolic agents. However, because the data have been conflicting, fluoride has not been approved by the FDA for treatment of osteoporosis. More data to prove fracture efficacy and safety of fluoride are needed.

Growth Hormone and IGF-1

Growth hormone is essential for both the acquisition of and maintenance of the skeleton. Many of the effects of growth hormone are mediated through another hormone, IGF-1, also known as somatomedin-C. Growth hormone deficiency in childhood is associated with short stature and low bone mass.[45] It is possible that the effect of growth hormone deficiency on BMD in children could be due to delayed puberty and insufficient gonadal steroids rather than to a direct effect of growth hormone or IGF-1. Alternatively, the low bone mass seen in growth hormone–deficient children could also be due to a direct effect of growth hormone or IGF-1 deficiency on growing bone. Preliminary data suggest that there is an increased risk of vertebral fracture in growth hormone–deficient adults. Lower bone density and increased fracture risk in these individuals could result from failure to achieve adequate peak adult bone mass rather than from reduced bone formation or increased bone resorption secondary to current growth hormone deficiency. No effect has been shown on hip fractures to date, but this may be due to a lack of appropriately sized studies. Observational data suggest that human growth hormone treatment for pituitary patients with growth hormone deficiency decreases fracture risk.[46]

Because of the known effects of growth hormone on bone acquisition, growth hormone and IGF-1 have been proposed as anabolic therapies for osteoporosis. Growth hormone can directly stimulate bone remodeling and increase endochondral growth through its actions on the osteoblast. Administration of growth hormone results in an increase in osteocalcin and, to a lesser extent, bone-specific alkaline phosphatase, suggesting an effect on bone formation.[47] Most studies that used growth hormone have shown only a very small increase in bone mass with therapy; one study by Rosen et al[48] even reported a decrease in BMD after 1 year of growth hormone in frail elderly men and women, despite an increase in osteocalcin and serum IGF-1. In the Rosen study, osteocalcin and NTx both increased to the same extent, suggesting a balanced increase in bone turnover, not just bone formation. Most studies have been 2 years or less in length, and it is possible that the lack of observed effect is due to the short duration of these trials.[49,50] One study,[51] in which growth hormone was added to ongoing estrogen therapy in postmenopausal women, showed no effect at 3 years, but by 4 years there was a statistically significant 14% increase in lumbar spine bone mass, and this benefit was maintained through the end of the 5-year study.

A 2-year trial of growth hormone administration in men showed an increase in BMD at both the lumbar spine and the total body after just 2 years.[52] Growth hormone was stopped after 2 years, and the men were followed for another year. One year after growth hormone was discontinued, there was a further increase in bone density at both the spine and the total body in this group of men.

Side effects related to growth hormone therapy include weight gain, edema, glucose intolerance, and carpal tunnel syndrome. Most of the effects of growth hormone occur through IGF-1. Hypothetically, IGF-1 could be clinically superior to growth hormone, because it stimulates bone formation more directly. In theory, this might lead to fewer side effects. However, IGF-1 has effects on many organ systems and could potentially have yet-undiscovered serious side effects as well.

Studies have suggested that serum IGF-1 levels are related to bone density in both men and women[53,54] and that low levels of IGF-1 may be associated with greater risk of hip and spine fractures.[55] With IGF-1 therapy, osteocalcin seems to increase more than deoxypyridinoline, suggesting an increase in overall bone turnover but a preferential effect on bone formation.[47]

Longer studies examining fracture data with both growth hormone and IGF-1 are needed to establish them as safe and effective anabolic agents.

Strontium

Strontium is a divalent cation that is closely chemically related to calcium. It has been shown to increase bone-specific alkaline phosphatase and to decrease urinary NTx, suggesting that it may both increase bone formation and decrease bone resorption. An increase in BMD at the lumbar spine has been observed after administration of strontium ranelate, and, at the higher dose of 2 g/day, a decreased risk for new vertebral fractures was reported.[56,57] Bone biopsy specimens showed normal mineralization of bone with no change in bone crystallization (as was seen with fluoride). Strontium thus far seems to be a promising and well-tolerated agent, but further research regarding fracture reduction efficacy and safety needs to be done.

3-Hydroxy-3-Methylglutaryl Coenzyme A Reductase Inhibitors

Several lines of evidence have suggested that the 3-hydroxy-3-methylglutaryl coenzyme A (HMG CoA) reductase inhibitors (statins) may also have an anabolic effect on bone. In 1999, Mundy et al[58] reported that the statins activated the bone morphogenic protein-2 (BMP-2) gene promoter. The BMP-2 gene was selected because it was known to increase osteoblast differentiation. Mundy's group also showed increased bone formation in murine calvarial bones after exposure to statins.

After this work with animal models, several population studies reported a decrease in fracture risk in patients on HMG CoA reductase inhibitors, although results of these observational studies have not been uniform. Most of them show a significant reduction in vertebral and hip fracture risk in patients taking statins,[59–63] but at least one trial showed no effect of statins on fracture risk.[64] Unfortunately, these are all observational studies with the biases inherent in this type of research.

The nitrogen-containing bisphosphonates, alendronate and risedronate, and the statins both inhibit steps in the cholesterol biosynthetic pathway. The statins inhibit HMG CoA reductase, the rate-limiting step in cholesterol biosynthesis. The bisphosphonates inhibit farnesyl pyrophosphate synthase, a step further down in the cholesterol synthetic pathway. Inhibiting the pathway at this point blocks the formation of proteins required for osteoclast function.

Because of the frequency of statin use and the prevalence of osteoporosis, it is important that RCTs be done to evaluate the efficacy of statins in decreasing osteoporotic fracture risk.

Summary

At the current time, the only FDA-approved anabolic agent for osteoporosis is hPTH (1-34). However, many exciting medications are being studied at this time and, hopefully, we will have a choice of anabolic agents and antiresorptive agents for treatment of osteoporosis in the near future.

Combination Therapy

It is inherent in the clinical practice of medicine that when a physician believes a patient is "nonresponding" or has less than an adequate response to the current therapy, either the therapy is changed, or combination (2 or more) therapies that may have different mechanisms of action to achieve the same clinical end point are considered.

For example, in the treatment of hypertension, combination therapies are often used to lower the blood pressure to the desired level. Although this clinical management approach seems plausible in the treatment of postmenopausal osteoporosis (PMO), the situation is not so clear-cut as it may be in the management of hypertension. This is because the surrogate end points currently used to monitor drug efficacy in the treatment of PMO, changes in BMD, or changes in the biochemical markers of bone turnover (BCM) are imperfect surrogates. That is, patients who have no increase in BMD may still have a reduction in fracture risk in the treated group compared with the placebo group who lose BMD; and the reductions in the BCM of bone resorption seen with antiresorptive agents account for only a small portion of the reduction in fracture risk (Fig. 7-9).[65–67] Furthermore, there are small changes in resorption markers with raloxifene yet substantial reductions in incident vertebral fractures. Finally, none of the current therapeutic agents used to treat

Figure 7-9. The relationship between changes in BMD and changes in vertebral fracture incidence. (Data from Nancollas GH, Tang R, Gulde S, et al: Mineral binding affinities and zeta potentials of biphosphonates. J Bone Miner Res 17(S1):5368, 2002.)

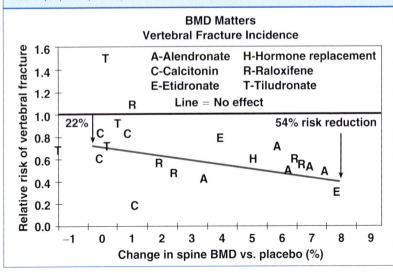

PMO abolishes fracture risk. Thus, a new vertebral fracture that occurs in a patient on any of the current agents used for the treatment of PMO may not indicate a therapeutic nonresponse. The greater the number of risk factors for fracture, the greater the risk for incident fracture.[68] Hence, high-risk patients may still fracture, even though they are having a positive bone biologic effect of the specific osteoporosis pharmacologic agent. Yet, most clinicians, when confronted with a patient who is adherent to therapy yet continues to fracture or lose BMD on therapy without an identifiable secondary medical cause, consider adding a second therapeutic agent. What is the evidence that combination therapies for the treatment of PMO have any advantage over a single agent? What is the evidence for better efficacy on the basis of BMD changes as opposed to fracture benefit? In addition, whereas the initial data on combination therapy combined two antiresorptive agents (estrogen or raloxifene with a bisphosphonate), with the recent introduction of intermittent parathyroid hormone (teriparatide), we need to examine the impact teriparatide will have in patients previously exposed to an antiresorptive agent vs. the teriparatide pivotal trial in which teriparatide-treated patients had not had previous exposure to a different pharmacologic agent.

No data exist on the effect of combination therapies on fracture risk reduction; thus, the data discussed are the effects of combination therapy on BMD and BCM of bone turnover. To the extent that these surrogates are associated to some degree of the magnitude of fracture risk reduction, the evidence for risk reduction is based on indirect associations.[65–67]

Combination therapy for postmenopausal osteoporosis was first examined with patients previously on ERT (conjugated equine estrogen, Premarin), 0.625 mg/day, or an equivalent estrogen dose recommended by the manufacturer for the management of osteoporosis.[69] Patients were assigned to continue their ERT alone (prior average duration of use, 9 years) or had alendronate, 10 mg/day, added to their ERT. The data suggest that even in postmenopausal women previously exposed to ERT, the addition of alendronate added an additional significant increase in spine and hip BMD, as opposed to continuation of ERT without adding this alternate antiresorptive agent. Although the magnitude of increase in BMD in the estrogen-alendronate group was greater than the BMD changes in the ERT group alone, the changes in BMD in the combination group were less than those reported in previous trials of estrogen and alendronate monotherapy. Similar data have also been shown with combinations of estrogen and etidronate.[70] Thus, it is possible that prior exposure to estrogen blunted a BMD response that might be expected to be greater in previously untreated patients. The scientific study that has compared combination therapy (ERT plus bisphosphonates) with previously untreated postmenopausal women is the observations by Bone et al.[71] In this study, 425 hysterectomized postmenopausal women without previous osteoporosis-specific pharmacologic therapy who had a mean T score of −2.5 were randomly assigned to receive either conjugated equine estrogen (0.625 mg/day), alendronate (10 mg/day), or combination therapy with both compounds for 2 years. The combined-treatment group (Fig 7-10) had a significantly greater increase in spine and femoral

Figure 7-10. Effect of estrogen replacement therapy, alendronate, or combinations of both on BMD in previously untreated postmenopausal women. (Data from Bone HG, Greenspan SL, McKeever C, et al: Alendronate and estrogen effects in postmenopausal women with low bone mineral density. J Clin Endocrinol Metab 85:720–726, 2000.) *(Continued on next page.)*

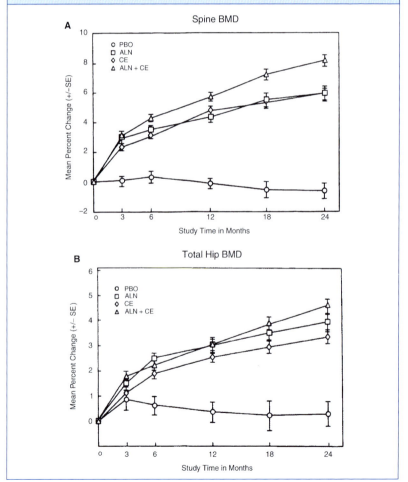

neck BMD than the increase in BMD seen by either estrogen or alendronate alone. In addition, the reduction in the biochemical marker of bone resorption, NTX, was also greater in the combined-treatment group as opposed to either single-treatment group. Furthermore, quantitative double-tetracycline–labeled bone histomorphometry was performed on 98 patients who received at least 18 months of treatment. There was a significantly lower mineralizing surface (%) between the combined-treatment group and placebo or either single-treatment groups, consistent with a greater suppression of bone turnover with the combined use of two different antiresorptive agents. Once again, this study was not powered for an analysis of fracture reduction differences, so it is unknown

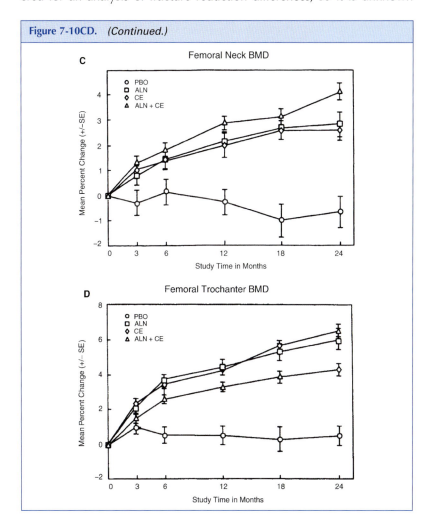

Figure 7-10CD. *(Continued.)*

whether the differences that were seen between the combined-treatment groups and the single-treatment groups translate into any differences in fracture risk reduction. It is also not known whether the reduction in bone turnover to the greater degree seen with combined therapy might, in the long run, suppress bone remodeling to the extent that repair of microdamage in normally stressed bone becomes impaired. Similar observations of the greater effect on BMD have been seen with estrogen alone vs. risedronate alone vs. combination therapy (Fig. 7-11).[72]

From a clinical point of view, this author does consider adding a bisphosphonate to ongoing ERT in four clinical scenarios:

1. Patients fracturing on ERT without an identifiable secondary cause.

2. Patients losing BMD on ERT without an identifiable secondary cause.

3. Patients with persistently elevated NTX on ERT without an identifiable secondary cause.

4. Patients with BMD hip T scores <−2.5 who are elderly and, therefore, have an increased risk for hip fracture.

Figure 7-11. Effect of estrogen or risedronate alone and in combination on BMD in postmenopausal women. (Data from Harris ST, Eriksen EF, Davidson M, et al: Effect of combined risedronate and hormone replacement therapies on bone mineral density in postmenopausal women. J Clin Endocrinol Metab 86:1890–1897, 2001.)

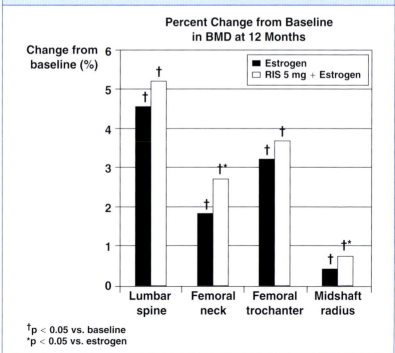

$^†p < 0.05$ vs. baseline
$^*p < 0.05$ vs. estrogen

Although ERT has just recently been shown to reduce the incidence of clinical vertebral fractures and hip fractures in the Women's Health Initiative (WHI) dataset, the fracture reduction was a secondary, not primary end point and from the perspective of FDA registration does not have a registration for the treatment of postmenopausal osteoporosis.[22] Hence, for women who continue to have the clinical bone associated with the scenarios previously described, this author will add a bisphosphonate, because the bisphosphonates have registrations for the reduction of vertebral, nonvertebral, and hip fracture risk. In addition, after withdrawal of estrogen, which is advised by many governmental and professional societies in light of the WHI negative cardiovascular risk findings, there is an accelerated bone loss, whereas there is not an accelerated bone loss after the withdrawal of alendronate or combination therapy of estrogen and bisphosphonate (Fig. 7-12).[73] This observation is most likely due to the different mechanism(s) of action of estrogen as opposed to bisphosphonate on bone. Although estrogen's effect is predominantly a cellular one, bisphosphonates mechanism of action on

Figure 7-12. The effect of discontinuation of estrogen or alendronate on BMD in postmenopausal women. (Data from Greenspan SL, Emkey RD, Bone H III, et al. Significant differential effects of alendronate, estrogen, or combination therapy on the rate of bone loss after discontinuation of treatment of post-menopausal osteoporosis. Ann Intern Med 137:875–883, 2002.)

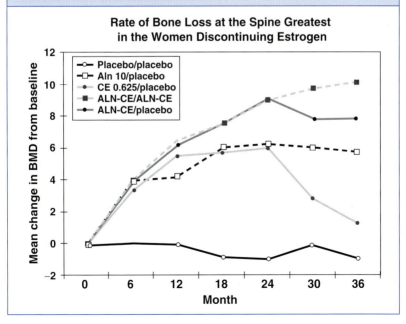

bone is both cellular and physiochemical. With the physiochemical and bone–binding mechanism of bisphosphonates action being a prolonged one, bisphosphonates maintain BMD after discontinuation longer than estrogen. In light of these observations of a rapid decline in BMD and an increase in fractures in the first year after estrogen withdrawal, physicians need to consider bisphosphonates after withdrawal of ERT.[74]

There are data for combinations of raloxifene with bisphosphonates as well.[75] In postmenopausal women started on raloxifene compared with alendronate compared with combinations of raloxifene and alendronate together, there is a greater increase in BMD with combination therapy as opposed to single therapy alone. Again, there are no fracture data to document that the greater increase in BMD with combination therapy translates into greater risk reduction.

With the recent FDA registration of teriparatide for the treatment of PMO and male osteoporosis and with the FDA label that suggests that teriparatide be used for "high-risk" patients, many patients will have teriparatide added to ongoing antiresorptive therapy. Although the pivotal clinical trial that led to the FDA registration of teriparatide randomly assigned previously untreated patients, there will be a need for data to see what the effect of teriparatide has on BMD and fracture risk reduction in patients either previously exposed to or on concomitant antiresorptive therapy. Although many of these combination clinical trials are currently underway, there are some data to suggest that prior exposure to an antiresorptive agent may mitigate at least the BMD or bone formation marker response to teriparatide.

In patients previously treated with ERT, several trials have examined the effect of adding PTH to patients who continued ERT as opposed to patients who continued ERT but did not receive PTH.[37,76] These trials showed significant increases in spinal BMD similar to the magnitude of increase in BMD seen in the teriparatide pivotal trial of patients who had never been exposed to ERT (Fig. 7-13). These comparisons are not head-to-head, and, in addition, in the combination trials just cited, there was no PTH-only arm. Yet, the rise in BMD with combinations of ERT and PTH was quite large, suggesting that the prior exposure to this specific antiresorptive agent might not blunt a subsequent response to PTH. In addition, data on patients on chronic glucocorticoid therapy for rheumatologic diseases and ERT demonstrated two important observations: PTH increased BMD while the patients maintained ERT and glucocorticoids, whereas the ERT-only group on glucocorticoids maintained BMD; and, second, when PTH was discontinued, BMD was maintained at the previously PTH-mediated higher level (Fig. 7-14).[76] This latter observation is important, because preliminary data suggest that unless an antiresorptive agent is used after discontinuing PTH, the PTH-mediated gain in BMD will be lost.[38,39]

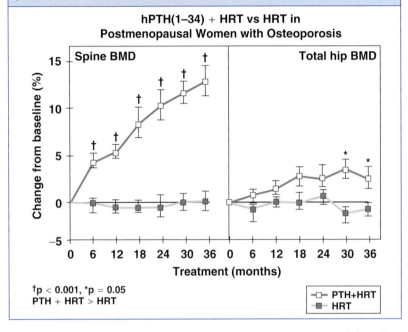

Figure 7-13. Effects of adding parathyroid hormone to ongoing estrogen replacement therapy vs. continuation of estrogen on BMD in postmenopausal women. (Data from Lindsay R, Nieves J, Formica C, et al: Randomised controlled study of effect of parathyroid hormone on vertebral-bone mass and fracture incidence among postmenopausal women on estrogen with osteoporosis. Lancet 350 (9077):550–555, 1997.)

Recent preliminary data that represent an interim analysis of the effect of PTH in patients previously exposed to alendronate or raloxifene have been reported.[77-79] Prior short-term (6 months) exposure to alendronate adding PTH or simultaneous combining of alendronate with PTH was completed in two studies. Combination therapy seemed to mitigate the bone formation marker response vs. PTH alone; PTH alone appeared to increase cortical bone volume (bone size) more than either alendronate alone or combination therapy. The increase in spine BMD seen with the combined therapy was similar to the PTH alone and much greater than the alendronate-alone group. The hip BMD increase was greater with the combined therapy than the change in hip BMD seen with PTH or alendronate alone. In the raloxifene interim analysis dataset, patients received either raloxifene (60 mg/day) or alendronate (10 mg/day) for 18 months and then the antiresorptive was discontinued while teriparatide was added for 12 months. Although the spine and hip BMD increased more in those patients previously treated with raloxifene at month 6, by the 12th month of PTH there were no differences in hip BMD between groups; and the

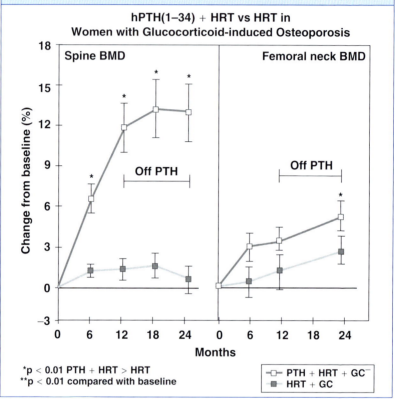

Figure 7-14. Effect of adding and then stopping parathyroid hormone on BMD in patients also receiving estrogen replacement therapy, as well as chronic glucocorticoid therapy. (Data from Finkelstein J, Hayes A, Rao A, et al: Effects of parathyroid hormone, alendronate, or both on bone density in osteoporotic men. J Bone Miner Res 17 (Suppl. 1): S127 (1007), 2002.)

slope of the increase in spine BMD in patients previously treated with alendronate was the same as raloxifene pre-treated patients from month 6 to month 12 of PTH treatment. It is important to stress that these datasets are preliminary and interim. Larger prospective data are needed to understand the impact of combining teriparatide with any antiresorptive agent and whether continuing or discontinuing the antiresorptive agent when teriparatide is added is a better choice. Furthermore, it is possible that differences will be seen when teriparatide is added to different bis-phosphonates because of the different bone affinities between aminobis-phosphonates.

At present, the use of combination therapies is based more on clinical judgment than scientific data. Even though greater BMD increases may be seen with combination therapy, it is unknown whether these

Table 7-4.	The Future of Osteoporosis Therapies

Shorter-acting inhibitors of bone resorption: osteoprotegerin, anti-rank-ligand antibody, integrins, prostaglandins

Anabolic agents: prostaglandins, strontium, 1-84 PTH, PTHrp, androgen receptor modulators, human growth hormone, IGF-1

Alternative selective estrogen receptor modulators (SERMS)

Isoflavones

Vitamin D metabolites

ANGELs

Gene therapy

BMD changes translate into better fracture risk reduction than can be achieved with monotherapy alone.

Future Directions

The future of pharmacologic therapy for osteoporosis is bright (Table 7-4). Newer and shorter-acting antiresorptive agents are either in clinical trials or in phase I or phase II development. These newer antiresorptive molecules may alter osteoclast function with a much shorter biologic half-life ($T\frac{1}{2}$) than current agents, especially the bisphosphonates. We have come to understand that there are differences within the aminobisphosphonate class, some of which have to do with the affinity and/or bone residence time of bisphosphonates. Hence, long-term safety, while at present not of any great concern, could become an issue as bisphosphonates are used for many years. Antiresorptive agents that do not have long residence time(s) in human tissue would be attractive.

Shorter-Acting Antiresorptives: Osteoprotegerin (OPG), Cathepsin K Inhibitors, Integrins, and Prostaglandins

Osteoprotegerin (OPG), the integrins, various prostaglandin derivatives, and other molecules that modulate the rank, rank-ligand, and OPG system will offer the ability to affect osteoclastic bone resorption with molecules that have short duration of activity and are not stored in human tissue.[80–84] Figure 7-15 shows how the osteoblast-derived OPG or rank-ligand may compete for the osteoclast-located receptor, rank. OPG (a rank "dummy"), which is given in the current phase III clinical trials by subcutaneous (SQ) injection, inhibits osteoclast activity by preventing rank-ligand from binding to its receptor, rank.

Although integrin and prostaglandin development is in early phases, they too may offer means of inhibiting osteoclast-mediated bone resorption. The ubiquitous receptor location and various affinities for receptor

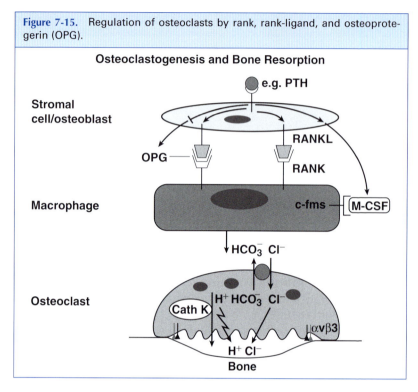

Figure 7-15. Regulation of osteoclasts by rank, rank-ligand, and osteoprotegerin (OPG).

binding that exist for these two different agents are the limitations of development. Yet the science by which these two can affect osteoclasts is of enough interest to sustain continual investigation.

Cathepsin K is an osteoclast-mediated product that is needed to help degrade type I bone collagen. Anti-cathepsin K molecules are in early phase I and phase II clinical development programs exploring their potential as inhibitors of bone resorption.[85,86]

For the anabolic agents, data have recently been presented suggesting that strontium, which stimulates osteoblasts and may also reduce osteoclast activities, may reduce both vertebral and nonvertebral fractures in postmenopausal women.[87] Other peptide sequences of PTH (1-84) and PTH-like compounds (PTHrp) may offer the ability to increase osteoblast function, the latter possibly without inducing hypercalcemia.[88,89]

One of the inherent difficulties with modifying the remodeling space and the remodeling unit is the inherent coupling between osteoclast and osteoblast function. In all the current pharmacologic therapeutic approaches to osteoporosis, whenever one decreases (or increases) the activity of one cell line, the change in the same direction occurs in the other cell line. Thus, whenever an antiresorptive agent reduces bone resorption by inhibiting osteoclast differentiation or function, in time, there will also be a reduction in osteoblast function. Likewise, whenever osteoblast function is increased (as it is with teriparatide), there will be an ensuing increase in osteoclast function. Thus, all the current osteoporosis therapies are limited in their effect by the natural linkage that exists between these two cell lines. In the future, various combinations or sequences of antiresorptive and anabolic agents may allow the coupling to become, for some time, "uncoupled" to facilitate a greater increase in BMD or modulation of bone microarchitecture in a more favorable way on bone strength.

The most abundant cell in bone is the osteocyte, a cell whose function has, heretofore, been altered by mechanical changes in bone.[90,91] Mechanical strain on bone tissue is a stimulus to osteocyte function, which, in turn, increases bone strength (mechano-stat) in animal models. Pharmacologic manipulation of the osteocyte is only a preliminary stage of bone research. More recently, the osteocyte has been shown to be negatively affected by glucocorticoids (glucocorticoids induce osteocyte apoptosis, and they do the same for osteoblasts) and that aminobisphosphonates mitigate this osteocyte and osteoblast effect, thereby increasing the pool of osteocytes and osteoblasts in the setting of glucocorticoids.[92,93] Thus, there is evidence that bisphosphonates (and more recently teriparatide) affect osteocyte function, leading to the possibility that the future may reveal how such alteration(s) change bone strength and reduce fracture risk (which might, in part, be independent of changes in BMD or turnover).[94,95]

Newer SERMS that may have greater effects on BMD and fewer side effects (such as hot flushes) are in development. Two such agents, lasofoxifene and BZA, are in phase III clinical trials, with only very preliminary evidence available.[96–98]

In addition, newer intravenous bisphosphonates, ibandronate and zoledronic acid, may offer the means to ensure bisphosphonate delivery to bone without any gastrointestinal risk exposure. In addition, the less frequent dosing (every 2-3 months with ibandronate and possibly once a year with zoledronic acid) may be appealing to patients and clinicians alike. The tight affinity of binding to bone seen with zolendronic acid caused by the presence of affinity-determining two nitrogen groups must be explored in greater detail so we know whether annual or less often dosing is needed.[14,99]

ANGELs (activators of non-genomic estrogen ligands) is a new paradigm of biology that is being investigated.[100] The paradigm thesis is that there is a nongenomic pathway of sex-steroid action in contrast to all our current knowledge suggesting that sex-steroid mechanisms of action are through genomic pathways. This nongenomic pathway may not even be sex-steroid specific, at least in mature bone cells. ANGELs may be powerfully agonistic in bone but have no effect on mammary or uterine tissue. It is unknown whether ANGELs affect the hypothalamic-pituitary-gonadal axis, a key area. Nevertheless, ANGELs may be an entirely new approach to modulation of bone tissue.

Human Growth Hormone (HGH)

In the 1990s, recombinant human growth hormone (rhGH) was approved by the FDA as "replacement" therapy for growth hormone deficiency on the basis of solid data that rhGH increased both muscle and bone mass in this specific population.[101] Clinical trials in patients without growth hormone deficiency have been discouraging, with little to no effect on BMD.[46] These unimpressive observations plus epidemiologic data suggesting that IGF-1 levels (which increase in response to rhGH administration) are associated with increased risk of prostate, breast, and colon cancer dissuaded any further investigative work into rhGH for osteoporosis.[102] However, most recently, data using a different dosing schedule in postmenopausal women who were maintained on estrogen, impressive increases in bone mineral content (BMC) and

---

Key Points: Pharmacologic Treatment of Osteoporosis

↣ The goal of therapy for osteoporosis is to prevent fractures.

↣ Pharmacologic interventions for osteoporosis fall into two main categories: antiresorptive agents and anabolic agents.

↣ The antiresorptive agents currently approved by the FDA have all been shown to increase bone mass and to decrease the risk of vertebral fractures; only the oral bisphosphonates, alendronate and risedronate, have been reported to also decrease the risk of hip fractures.

↣ The only anabolic agent currently approved by the FDA is teriparatide, which has been shown to increase bone mass and to reduce the risk of both vertebral and nonvertebral fractures; specific hip fracture prevention efficacy has not yet been evaluated with an adequately powered clinical trial.

↣ Combination therapies with two antiresorptive agents in general suppress bone turnover to a greater extent than monotherapy.

↣ Combination therapies with two antiresorptive agents in general increase BMD to a slightly greater extent than monotherapy.

↣ Combination therapy with an antiresorptive agent and an anabolic agent might not mitigate the anabolic agents effect on BMD.

↣ There are no fracture data with regard to the effect of combination therapy on fracture risk.

BMD have been seen along with increases in lean body mass, which could offer secondary benefits for fall reduction in the elderly.[51] Hence, there may be a resurgence of interest in reexamining the potential for rhGH in the treatment of osteoporosis.[50]

The future is bright for many research and clinical opportunities in osteoporosis and in the clinical development programs. Because osteoporosis of many etiologies and in both genders is an important clinical and public health issue, newer developments are certainly promising.

References

1. Black DM, Cummings SR, Karpf DB, et al, for the Fracture Intervention Trial Research Group: Randomised trial of effect of alendronate on risk of fracture in women with existing vertebral fractures. Lancet 348:1535–1541, 1996.
2. Tonino RP, Meunier PJ, Emkey R, et al, for the Phase III Osteoporosis Treatment Study Group: Skeletal benefits of alendronate: 7-year treatment of postmenopausal osteoporotic women. J Clin Endocrinal Metab 85:3109–3115, 2000.
3. Bone HG, Hosking D, Devogelaer JP, et al: Ten-years experience with alendronate for osteoporosis in postmenopausal women. N Engl J Med 350:1189–1199, 2004.
4. The Osteoporosis Methodology Group, The Osteoporosis Research Advisory Group. Meta-analyses of therapies for postmenopausal osteoporosis. Endocr Rev 23:496–507, 2002.
5. Schnitzer T, Bone HG, Crepaldi G, for the Alendronate once-weekly study group: Therapeutic equivalence of alendronate 70 mg once-weekly and alendronate 10 mg daily in the treatment of osteoporosis. Aging Clin Exp Res 12:1–12, 2000.
6. Harris ST, Watts NB, Genant HK, et al: for the Vertebral Efficacy With Risedronate Therapy (VERT) Study Group. Effects of risedronate treatment on vertebral and nonvertebral fractures in women with postmenopausal osteoporosis. JAMA 282:1344–1352, 1999.
7. Reginster JY, Minne HW, Sorensen OH, et al, for the Vertebral Efficacy With Risedronate Therapy (VERT) Study Group: Randomized trial of the effects of risedronate on vertebral fractures in women with established postmenopausal osteoporosis. Osteoporos Int 11:83–91, 2000.
8. Sorensen OH, Crawford GM, Mulder H, et al: Long-term efficacy of risedronate: a 5-year placebo-controlled clinical experience. Bone 32:120–126, 2003.
9. McClung MR, Geusens P, Miller PD, for the Hip Intervention Program Study Group: Effect of risedronate on the risk of hip fracture in elderly women. N Engl J Med 344:333–340, 2001.
10. Brown JP, Kendler DL, McClung MR, et al: The efficacy and tolerability of risedronate once a week for the treatment of postmenopausal osteoporosis. Calcif Tissue Int 71:103–111, 2002.
11. Storm T, Thamsborg G, Steiniche T, et al: Effect of intermittent cyclical etidronate therapy on bone mass and fracture rate in women with postmenopausal osteoporosis. N Engl J Med 322:1265–1271, 1990.
12. Watts NB, Harris ST, Genant HK, et al: Intermittent cyclical etidronate treatment of postmenopausal osteoporosis. N Engl J Med 323:73–79, 1990.
13. Thiebaud D, Burckhardt P, Melchior J, et al: Two years' effectiveness of intravenous pamidronate (APD) versus oral fluoride for osteoporosis occurring in the postmenopause. Osteoporos Int 4(2):76–83, 1994.

14. Reid IR, Brown JP, Burckhardt P, et al: Intravenous zoledronic acid in postmenopausal women with low bone mineral density. N Engl J Med 346:653–661, 2002.
15. Thiebaud D, Burckhardt P, Kriegbaum H, et al: Three monthly intravenous injections of ibandronate in the treatment of postmenopausal osteoporosis. Am J Med 103(4):298–307, 1997.
16. Ettinger B, Black DM, Mitlak BH, et al: for the Multiple Outcomes of Raloxifene Evaluation (MORE) Investigators. Reduction of vertebral fracture risk in post-menopausal women with osteoporosis treated with raloxifene. Results from a 3-year randomized clinical trial. JAMA 282:637–645, 1999.
17. Maricic M, Adachi J, Sarkar S, et al: Early effects of raloxifene on clinical vertebral fractures at 12 months in postmenopausal women with osteoporosis. Am J Med 162:1140–1143, 2002.
18. Delmas PD, Ensrud KE, Adachi JD, et al: Efficacy of raloxifene on vertebral fracture risk reduction on postmenopausal women with osteoporosis: four year results from a randomized controlled trial. J Clin Endocrinol Metab 87: 3609–3617, 2002.
19. Cummings SR, Eckert S, Krueger KA, et al: The effect of raloxifene on risk of breast cancer in postmenopausal women. Results from the MORE randomized trial. JAMA 281:2189–2197, 1999.
20. Barrett-Connor E, Grady D, Sashegyi A, et al, for the MORE Investigators: Raloxifene and cardiovascular events in osteoporotic postmenopausal women. Four-year results from the MORE (multiple outcomes of raloxifene evaluation) randomized trial. JAMA 287:847–857, 2002.
21. Chestnut III CH, Silverman S, Andriano K, et al: A randomized trial of nasal spray salmon calcitonin in postmenopausal women with established osteoporosis: the prevent recurrence of osteoporotic fractures study. PROOF study group. Am J Med 109(4): 267–276, 2000.
22. Writing Group for the Women's Health Initiative Investigators: Risk and benefits of estrogen plus progestin in healthy postmenopausal women. Principal results from the women's health initiative randomized controlled trial. JAMA 288:321–333, 2002.
23. Hulley S, Grady D, Bush T, et al: Randomized trial of estrogen plus progestin for second-ary prevention of coronary heart disease in postmenopausal women. Heart and estro-gen/progestin replacement study (HERS) research group. JAMA 280(7):605–613, 1998.
24. Grady D, Herrington D, Bittner V, et al, for the HERS Research Group: Cardiovascular disease outcomes during 6.8 years of hormone therapy. Heart and estrogen/progestin replacement study follow-up (HERS II). JAMA 288:49–57, 2002.
25. Hulley S, Furberg C, Barrett-Connor E, et al, for the HERS Research Group: Non-cardiovascular disease outcomes during 6.8 years of hormone therapy. Heart and estrogen/progestin replacement study follow-up (HERS II). JAMA 288:58–66, 2002.
26. Hays J, Ockene JK, Brunner RL, et al, for the Women's Health Initiative Investigators: Effects of estrogen plus progesterone on health-related quality of life. N Engl J Med 348:1839–1854, 2003.
27. Rapp SR, Espeland MA, Shumaker SA, et al: Effect of estrogen plus progestin on global cognitive function in postmenopausal women: the Women's Health Initiative Memory Study: a randomized controlled trial. JAMA 289:2663–2672, 2003.
28. Shumaker SA, Legault C, Thal L, et al: Estrogen plus progestin and the incidence of demen-tia and mild cognitive impairment in postmenopausal women: the Women's Health Initiative Memory Study: a randomized controlled trial. JAMA 289:2651–2662, 2003.
29. Morabito N, Crisafulli A, Vergara C, et al: Effect of genistein and hormone-replacement therapy on bone loss in early postmenopausal women: a randomized double-blind placebo-controlled study. J Bone Miner Res 17:1904–1912, 2002.

30. Feldman D: Vitamin D, parathyroid hormone, and calcium: a complex regulatory network. Am J Med 107(6):637–639, 1999.
31. Nissenson RA: Parathyroid hormone and parathyroid hormone related protein. In Marcus R, Feldman D, Kelsey J. Osteoporosis, 2nd ed. San Diego, CA, Academic Press, pp 221–246.
32. Albright F, Aub JC, Bauer W: Hyperparathyroidism: a common and polymorphic condition as illustrated by seventeen proven cases from one clinic. JAMA 102:1276–1287, 1934.
33. Selye H: On the stimulation of new bone-formation with parathyroid extract and irradiated ergosterol. J Endocrinology 16:547–555, 1932.
34. Neer RM, Arnaud CD, Zanchetta JR, et al.: Effect of parathyroid hormone (1-34) on fractures and bone mineral density in postmenopausal women with osteoporosis. N Engl J Med 344:1434–1441, 2001.
35. Fujita T, Inoue T, Morii H, et al: Effect of an intermittent weekly dose of human parathyroid hormone (1–34) on osteoporosis: a randomized double-masked prospective study using three dose levels. Osteoporosis Int. 9:296–306, 1999.
36. Rittmaster RS, Bolognese M, Ettinger MP, et al: Enhancement of bone mass in osteoporotic women with parathyroid hormone followed by alendronate. J Clin Endocrinol Metab 85:2129–2134, 2000.
37. Lindsay R, Nieves J, Formica C, et al: Randomised controlled study of effect of parathyroid hormone on vertebral-bone mass and fracture incidence among postmenopausal women on estrogen with osteoporosis. Lancet 350 (9077):550–555, 1997.
38. Orwoll E, Scheele WH, Paul S, et al. The effect of teriparatide [human parathyroid hormone (1-34)] therapy on bone density in men with osteoporosis. J Bone Min Res 18:9–17, 2003.
39. Kurland ES, Cosman F, McMahon D, et al: Parathyroid hormone as a therapy for idiopathic osteoporosis in men: effects on bone mineral density and bone markers. J Clin Endocrinol Metab 85:3069–3076, 2000.
40. Vahle JL, Sato M, Long GG, et al: Skeletal changes in rats given daily subcutaneous injections of recombinant human parathyroid hormone (1-34) for 2 years and relevance to human safety. Toxicol Pathol 30(3):312–321, 2002.
41. Lau KHW, Baylink DJ: Molecular mechanism of action of fluoride on bone cells. J Bone Min Res 13:1660–1667, 1998.
42. Riggs BL, Hodgson SF, O'Fallon WM, et al: Effect of fluoride treatment on the fracture rate in postmenopausal women with osteoporosis. N Engl J Med 322:802–809, 1990.
43. Kleerekoper M, Peterson EL, Nelson DA, et al: A randomized trial of sodium fluoride as a treatment for postmenopausal osteoporosis. Osteoporos Int 1(3):155–161, 1991.
44. Pak CY, Sakhaee K, Adams-Huet B, et al: Treatment of postmenopausal osteoporosis with slow-release sodium fluoride: final report of a randomized controlled trial. Ann Intern Med 123:401–408, 1995.
45. Rosen CJ, Rackoff RJ: Emerging anabolic treatments for osteoporosis. Rheum Dis Clin NA 27:215–233, 2001.
46. Wuster C, Abs R, Bengtsson B-A, et al: The influence of growth hormone deficiency, growth hormone replacement therapy, and other aspects of hypopituitarism on fracture rate and bone mineral density. J Bone Miner Res 16:398–405, 2001.
47. Ghiron L, Thompson JL, Halloway L, et al: Effects of rhGH and IGF-1 on bone turnover in elderly women. J Bone Miner Res 10:1844–1852, 1995.
48. Rosen CJ, Friez J, MacLean D, et al: The RIGHT Study: a randomized placebo controlled trial of recombinant human growth hormone in frail elderly: dose response effects on bone mass and bone turnover. J Bone Miner Res 14:S208, 1999.

49. Rosen CJ, Bilezikian JP: Clinical review 123: HOT TOPIC: Anabolic therapy for osteoporosis. J Clin Endocrinol Metab 86:957–964, 2001.
50. Rosen CJ, Wuster C: Growth hormone rising: did we quit too quickly? J Bone Miner Res 18:406–409, 2003.
51. Landin-Wilhelmsen K, Nilsson A, Bosaeus I, et al: Growth hormone increases bone mineral content in postmenopausal osteoporosis: a randomized placebo-controlled trial. J Bone Miner Res 18:393–405, 2003.
52. Gillberg P, Mallmin H, Petrén-Mallmin, M, et al: Two Years of Treatment with Recombinant Human Growth Hormone Increases Bone Mineral Density in Men with Idiopathic Osteoporosis. J Clin Endocrinol Metab 87:4949–4956, 2002.
53. Celiker R, Arslan S: Comparison of serum insulin-like growth factor-1 and growth hormone levels in osteoporotic and non-osteoporotic postmenopausal women. Rheumatol Int 19(6):205–208, 2000.
54. Ljunghall S, Johansson AG, Burman K, et al: Low plasma levels of IGF-1 in male patients with idiopathic osteoporosis. J Intern Med 232:59–64, 1992.
55. Gamero P, Sornay-Rendu E, Delmas PD: Low serum IGF-1 and occurrence of osteoporotic fractures in postmenopausal women [letter]. Lancet 355(9207):898–899, 2000.
56. Reginster JY, Roux C, Tsouderos Y, et al: Role of strontium ranelate in prevention of early postmenopausal bone loss: a double-blind, prospective, randomised, placebo-controlled study. Arthritis Rheum 41(Suppl):S129(Abstract 580), 1998.
57. Meunier PJ, Slosman DO, Delmas PD, et al: Strontium ranelate: dose-dependent effects in established postmenopausal vertebral osteoporosis—a 2-year randomized placebo controlled trial. J Clin Endocrinol Metab 87:2060–2066, 2002.
58. Mundy G, Garrett R, Harris S, et al: Stimulation of bone formation in vitro and in rodents by statins. Science 286:1946–1949, 1999.
59. Chan KA, Andrade SE, Boles M: Inhibitors of hydroxymethylglutaryl-coenzyme A reductase and risk of fracture among older women. Lancet 355:2185–2188, 2000.
60. Chung Y, Lee M, Lee S, et al: HMG-CoA reductase inhibitors increase BMD in type 2 diabetes mellitus patients. J Clin Endocrinol Metab 85:1137–1142, 2000.
61. Meier CR, Schlienger RG, Kraenzlin ME, et al: HMG-CoA reductase inhibitors and the risk of fractures. JAMA 283:3205–3210, 2000.
62. Wang PS, Solomon DH, Mogun H, et al: HMG-CoA reductase inhibitors and the risk of hip fractures in elderly patients. JAMA 283:3211–3216, 2000.
63. Pasco JA, Kotowicz MA, Henry MJ, et al: Statin use bone mineral density, and fracture risk. Arch Intern Med 162:537–540, 2002.
64. van Staa T, Wegman S, de Vries F: Use of statins and risk of fractures. JAMA 285:1850–1855, 2001.
65. Wasnich RD, Miller PD: Antifracture efficacy of antiresorptive agents are related to changes in bone density. J Clin Endocrinol Metab 85:231–236, 2001.
66. Hochburg MC, Greenspan S, Wasnich RD, et al: Changes in bone density and turnover explain the reductions in incidence of non-vertebral fractures that occur during treatment with antiresorptive agents. J Clin Endocrinol Metab 87:1586–1592, 2002.
67. Cummings SR, Karpf DB, Harris F, et al: Improvements in spine bone density and reduction in risk of vertebral fractures during treatment with antiresorptive drugs. Am J Med 114:281–289, 2002.
68. Miller PD: Greater risk, greater benefit: true or false? J Clin Endocrinol Metab 88:538–541, 2003.
69. Lindsay R, Cosman F, Lobo RA, et al: Addition of alendronate to ongoing hormone replacement therapy in the treatment of osteoporosis: a randomized, controlled clinical trial. J Clin Endocrinol Metab 84:3076–3081, 1999.

70. Wimalawansa SJ: Combined therapy with estrogen and etidronate has an additive effect on bone mineral density in the hip and vertebrae: four year randomized study. Am J Med 99:36–42, 1995.
71. Bone HG, Greenspan SL, McKeever C, et al: Alendronate and estrogen effects in postmenopausal women with low bone mineral density. J Clin Endocrinol Metab 85:720–726, 2000.
72. Harris ST, Eriksen EF, Davidson M, et al: Effect of combined risedronate and hormone replacement therapies on bone mineral density in postmenopausal women. J Clin Endocrinol Metab 86:1890–1897, 2001.
73. Greenspan SL, Emkey RD, Bone H III, et al: Significant differential effects of alendronate, estrogen, or combination therapy on the rate of bone loss after discontinuation of treatment of postmenopausal osteoporosis. Ann Intern Med 137:875–883, 2002.
74. Barrett-Conner E, Wehren L, Siris E, et al: Recency and duration of postmenopausal hormone therapy: effects on bone mineral density and fracture risk in the National Osteoporosis Risk Assessment (NORA) study. Menopause 10:412–419, 2003.
75. Johnell O, Scheele WH, Reginster JY, et al: Additive effects of raloxifene and alendronate on bone density and biochemical markers of bone remodeling in postmenopausal women with osteoporosis. J Clin Endocrinol Metab 87:985–992, 2002.
76. Lane NE, Sanchez S, Modin GW, et al: Bone mass continues to increase at the hip after parathyroid treatment is discontinued in glucocorticoid induced osteoporosis: results of a randomized controlled clinical trial. J Bone Miner Res 15:944–951, 2000.
77. Finkelstein J, Hayes A, Rao A, et al: Effects of parathyroid hormone, alendronate, or both on bone density in osteoporotic men. N Engl J Med 349:1216–1226, 2003.
78. Neer R, Hayes A, Rao A, et al: Effects of parathyroid hormone, alendronate, or both on bone density in osteoporotic women. N Engl J Med 349:1207–1215, 2003.
79. Ettinger B, San Martin JA, Crans G, et al: Early response of bone turnover markers and bone mineral density to teriparatide [recombinant human parathyroid hormone (1-34)] in postmenopausal women previously treated with an antiresorptive drug. J Bone Min Res 18 (Suppl. 2):S15 (1053), 2003.
80. Hofbauer LC, Khosla S, Dunstan CR, et al: The roles of osteoprotegerin and osteoprotegerin ligand in the paracrine regulation of bone resorption. J Bone Miner Res 15:2–12, 2000.
81. Emery JG, McDonnell P, Burke MB, et al: OPG is a receptor for the cytokine ligand TRAIL. J Biol Chem 273:14363–14367, 1998.
82. Feng X, Novack DV, Faccio R, et al: A Glansmann's mutation in beta 3 integrin specifically impairs osteoclast function. J Clin Invest 107:1137–1144, 2001.
83. Weinreb M, Machwate M, Shir N, et al: Expression of the prostaglandin E2 (PGE2) receptor subtype EP4 and its regulation by PGE2 in osteoblastic cell lines and adult rat bone tissue. Bone 28:275–281, 2001.
84. Machwate M, Harada S, Leu CT, et al: Prostaglandin receptor EP(4) mediates the bone anabolic effects of PGE2. Mol Pharmacol 60: 36–41, 2001.
85. Rodan SB, Rodan GA: Function and regulation of cathepsin K in bone. Bone Key-Osteovision 1:1–5, 2001.
86. Kafienah W, Bromme D, Butte DJ, et al: Human cathepsin K cleaves native type I and II collagens at the N-terminal end of the triple helix. Biochem J 331:727–732, 1998.
87. Rubin MR, Bilezikian JP: New anabolic therapies in osteoporosis. Endocrinol Metab Clin North Am 32:285–307, 2003.
88. Parfitt AM: Perspective: parathyroid hormone and periosteal bone expansion. J Bone Miner Res 17:1741–1743, 2002.
89. Stewart AF: PTHrP (1-36) as a skeletal anabolic agent for the treatment of osteoporosis. Bone 19:303–306, 1996.

90. Marrotti G: The structure of bone tissues and the cellular control of their deposition. Ital J Anat Embryol 101:25–79, 1996.
91. Noble BS, Reeve J: Osteocyte function, osteocyte death and bone fracture resistance. Mol Cell Endocrinol 25:7–13, 2000.
92. Weinstein RS, Chen J-R, Powers CC, et al: Promotion of osteoclast survival and antagonism of bisphosphonate-induced osteoclast apoptosis by glucocorticoids. J Clin Invest 109:1041–1048, 2002.
93. Weinstein RS, Jilka RL, Parfitt M, et al: Inhibition of osteoblastogenesis and promotion of apoptosis of osteoblasts and osteocytes by glucocorticoids. J Clin Invest 102:274–282, 1998.
94. Manolagas SC: Corticosteroids and fractures: A close encounter of the third cell kind. J Bone Miner Res 15:1001–1005, 2000.
95. Zanchetta JR, Bogado CE, Ferretti JL, et al: Effects of teriparatide [recombinant human parathyroid hormone (1-34)] on cortical bone in postmenopausal women with osteoporosis. J Bone Miner Res 18:539–543, 2003.
96. Riggs BL, Hartmann LC: Selective estrogen-receptor-modulators—mechanisms of action and application to clinical practice. N Engl J Med 348:618–629, 2003.
97. Ke HZ, Qi H, Chidsey-Frink KL, et al: Lasofoxifene (CP-336,156) protects against the age-related changes in bone mass, bone strength, and total serum cholesterol in intact aged male rats. J Bone Miner Res 16:765–773, 2001.
98. Ronkin S, Clarke S, Boudes P, et al: TSE-424, a novel tissue selective estrogen, reduces biochemical indices of bone metabolism in a dose related fashion. J Bone Miner Res 16 (S1):S413, 2001.
99. Nancollas GH, Tang R, Gulde S, et al: Mineral binding affinities and zeta potentials of bisphosphonates. J Bone Miner Res 17(S1):S368, 2002.
100. Moggs JG, Deavall D, Orphanides G: Sex steroids, ANGELS, and osteoporosis. BioEssays 25:195–199, 2003.
101. Rudman D, Feller AG, Nagraj HS, et al: Effects of human growth hormone in men over 60 years old. N Engl J Med 323:1562–1563, 1990.
102. Chan JM, Stampfer MJ, Giovannucci E, et al: Plasma insulin-like growth factor–I and prostate cancer risk: a prospective study. Science 279:563–566, 1998.

Monitoring Osteoporosis Therapy

chapter

8

Paul D. Miller, M.D.

Monitoring Bone Mineral Density

The surrogate endpoint markers for monitoring the efficacy of osteoporosis-specific agents are changes in BMD and changes in biochemical markers (BCM) of bone turnover. Both of these surrogate markers have their proper place in clinical management, although neither is a perfect indicator of pharmacologic response or nonresponse to therapeutic interventions for antiresorptive agents.

The prevention or reduction of fractures is the ultimate goal of treatment. Yet, none of the osteoporosis-specific agents eliminate fracture risk. Hence, the occurrence of another (i.e., vertebral) fracture on antiresorptive agents does not necessarily mean that the patient has not had a pharmacologic effect of antiresorptive treatment. On the other hand, clinicians feel uncomfortable waiting for another fracture event to define treatment effectiveness; thus, clinicians use surrogate markers to assist their therapeutic strategies, analogous to lowering blood pressure or cholesterol to measure the treatment effect of antihypertensive or cholesterol-lowering agents as surrogates to measure efficacy to reduce heart attack risk.

The surrogate markers for osteoporosis-specific therapies are BMD and BCM of bone turnover, and there is increasing evidence for the latter's clinical application.[1] Because the most abundant data exist for changes in BMD and BCM with antiresorptive agents, the next section will emphasize these two surrogate markers for the antiresorptive agents. A few comments will be made about observed changes in BCM of bone turnover observed with the anabolic agent, intermittent parathyroid-hormone, teriparatide, just approved by the FDA in November 2002.

The BCM of bone formation that is most widely used is the bone-specific alkaline phosphatase (BSAP), and the BCMs of bone resorption that are most widely used in clinical practice are the collagen cross-links, N-telopeptide (NTX) and C-telopeptide (CTX), measured in urine or blood. Most clinicians in the United States are using urinary NTX, which is collected as a fasting, second-voided urine specimen.

It is insightful that even though the FDA's current requirement for registration of postmenopausal osteoporosis (PMO) -specific therapies still requires proof of a significant 3-year vertebral fracture reduction, the FDA has now approved both the once-a-week alendronate and the once-a-week risedronate formulations based not on any proven fracture benefit but on the evidence that these weekly formulations increase BMD and reduce BCM to equivalent degrees as the daily dosing. Hence, the FDA acknowledges that these two surrogate markers for these bisphosphonates explain the improvement in bone strength and the reduction in fracture incidence.

Because the once-a-week bisphosphonate registration has been done with no adequately powered preplanned fracture data, trust in these surrogate markers is the underpinning for confidence in drug effect of once-a-week formulations. Thus, these FDA registrations are based on the assumption that weekly dosing of bisphosphonates must be equivalent to daily dosing. Yet, to the extent that the "bone" half-life of bisphosphonates may not reflect the bone's biologic, functional bisphosphonate half-life and that the bone binding and alteration in activation-frequency of bisphosphonates differ between aminobisphosphonates, these assumptions may or may not be entirely valid.[2-5] In addition, there is evidence that bisphosphonates alter bone microarchitecture; in part, their improvement in bone strength might be unrelated to their capacity to improve BMD or reduce BCM and bone turnover.[6] Preservation of horizontal trabeculae as shown in Fig. 8-1 also increases bone strength. In this regard, publications have examined the relationship between the changes in BMD and/or BCM to the magnitude of reduction in either vertebral or nonvertebral incident fractures by robust meta-analysis of randomized controlled clinical trials (Figs. 8-2 and 8-3).[7-8] On balance, the two vertebral fracture meta-analyses are in agreement that a portion (24%–54%) of the risk reduction of antiresorptive agents can be attributed to the increase in BMD. These two meta-analyses agree that there is approximately a 24% reduction in vertebral fracture risk at the intercept (no change in BMD), indicating that other non-BMD mechanisms are playing a role in the improvement in bone strength. A comparison of these two meta-analyses shows they come to similar conclusions (Fig. 8–4). On the other hand, the meta-analysis of the relationships between the changes in BMD and BCM caused by antiresorptive agents and the reduction in *nonvertebral* fractures shows that all the effects of those antiresorptive

Figure 8-1. Preservation of horizontal trabeculae by the bisphosphonate, risedronate, in a minipig model. (Data from Borah B, Dufresne TE, et al: Risedronate preserves trabecular architecture and increases bone strength in vertebrae of ovariectomized minipigs as measured by three-dimensional microcomputed tomography. J Bone Miner Res 17:1139–1147, 2002.)

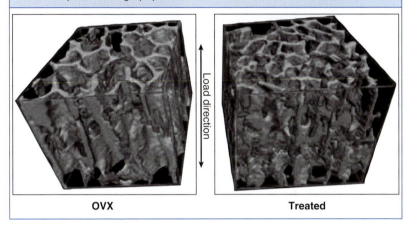

OVX   Treated

Figure 8-2. Greater increases in axial BMD are associated with greater reductions in vertebral fracture incidence. (Data from Wasnich RD, Miller PD: Antifracture efficacy of antiresorptive agents are related to changes in bone density. J Clin Endocrinol Metab 85:231–236, 2001.)

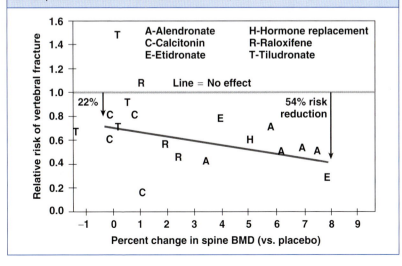

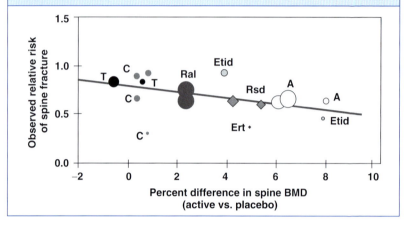

Figure 8-3. The association between the magnitude of increase in BMD and the greater reduction in vertebral fracture. (Data from Cummings SR, Karpf DB, Harris F, et al: Improvements in spine bone density and reduction in risk of vertebral fractures during treatment with antiresorptive drugs. Am J Med 114:281–289, 2002.)

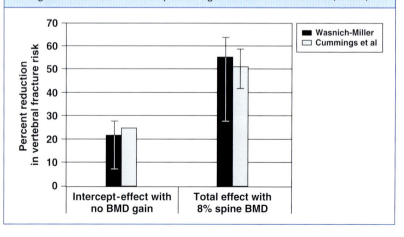

Figure 8-4. Similar conclusions of two separate meta-analyses showing the relationship in spinal BMD changes vs. no change in BMD and incident reduction in vertebral fractures. (Data from Wasnich RD, Miller PD: Antifracture efficacy of antiresorptive agents are related to changes in bone density. J Clin Endocrinol Metab 87:1586–1592, 2001; Cummings SR, Karpf DB, Harris F, et al: Improvements in spine bone density and reduction in risk of vertebral fractures during treatment with antiresorptive drugs. Am J Med 114:281–289, 2002.)

agents that reduce the incidence of nonvertebral fractures can be attributed to either the magnitude of increase in BMD or the magnitude of reduction in BCM of bone turnover.[9] In this meta-analysis, the risk reduction related to either the increase in BMD or the reduction in BCM could not be separated, because the adjusted variance that each component contributes to risk reduction is so similar that the two components cannot be distinguished.

Because the bisphosphonates are the only antiresorptive agents to show reductions in vertebral, nonvertebral, and hip fracture rates and are the only agents that produce the magnitude of increases in BMD in nonspine sites or magnitude of reduction in BCM that might be necessary to induce reductions in the risk of nonvertebral fractures, the recent meta-analyses cited provide evidence to support their therapeutic effect at nonvertebral sites. It simply may take greater increases in BMD and/or reductions of BCM to induce a reduction in nonvertebral fracture incidence than to induce a reduction in vertebral fracture incidence. Clearly, by reducing bone turnover, there could be microarchitectural changes in bone that might not be reflected in BMD measurements that lead to increased bone strength.

Alternately, the areal BMD measurements that we routinely use in bone densitometry could also be underestimating the real magnitude of BMD increases.[10-11] Areal BMD by DXA is a derived equation: BMD = BMC/area. The bone area could increase without any change or with a lesser change in BMC; thus the calculated BMD would decline, not necessarily because of any reduction in BMC but an increase in bone area. Evidence for this effect of bone area on calculated BMD comes from head-to-head studies measuring changes in areal BMD by DXA versus peripheral (forearm) quantitative computed tomography (pQCT), which measures the true bone mass in the teriparatide pivotal clinical trial.[12] Use of teriparatide showed increases in bone area both by pQCT and by three-dimensional microcomputed bone biopsy specimens.[13] In the cited PTH trial, BMC increased at the forearm as measured both by forearm DXA and forearm pQCT, yet calculated BMD by DXA declined while it increased by pQCT, indicating that areal BMD (DXA) measurements may underestimate the change in BMD when bone area also increases. Nevertheless, although areal BMD using DXA of the forearm declines in teriparatide-treated patients, bone strength improves at this skeletal site in teriparatide-treated patients because wrist fractures decline in treated as compared with untreated patients.

A few comments are pertinent regarding the challenge that serial BMD measurements may not adequately reflect changes in bone strength. Serial BMD has come under scrutiny as a means of monitoring therapy in patients receiving antiresorptive agents. Skepticism is more a function of the performance of the DXA measurement and the clinical interpretation.[14] For a clinician to know with certainty that a change in BMD between two measurements in an individual patient is real as opposed to an inherent measurement error of the DXA device or the technologist who is performing the test, the DXA site must do and then know their individual in vivo precision error.[15–17] Performing daily phantom (in vitro) scanning is important to detect a "drift" in serial BMD values that may indicate the need to obtain manufacturer assistance to examine issues that reflect machine performance: x-ray tube viability, soft-wear deterioration, etc. Yet, phantoms do not move, while patients do; for a DXA facility to really know whether differences are machine or biologic, in vivo precision studies must be completed. These are not difficult to do and allow a facility to know for certain whether a change in an individual patient is real or a machine/technologist measurement error.

There are published data on why and how to perform an in vivo precision study in a medical practice.[15,16] The basic principle is to know what your in vivo coefficient of variation % (CV%) is between multiple measurements, which then allows the physician to determine whether the difference between two measurements is within or beyond the least significant change (LSC). Without a DXA site knowing their independent precision error, changes in BMD may be assumed to be significant (or nonsignificant) when they may not be. For example, when the spine BMD goes up a small amount (~2%) and the total hip decreases (~4%), the DXA reports often state that the "patient is nonresponding," when in fact the precision error at the total hip even in the most exact DXA facilities is ~2%, requiring at least a 5.6% change in BMD to be significant. Many patients, unfortunately, are often taken off or have their therapies changed, because the BMD change is really within the LSC but misinterpreted to be significant. The densitometry community has set a standard requiring a 95% confidence limit to know whether a difference in two BMD measurements in an individual patient is significant or not. Within this definition, the change in BMD must be 2.77 × the CV% (precision error). Hence, it is evident that competent DXA sites must do in vivo precision studies to competently interpret BMD changes between two measurements. The simplest way to do a precision study is to do duplicate BMD scans on 30 patients and then do the calculations for the standard deviation of the measurements for each patient and then for the group, and then calculate the root mean square as well. The International Society for Clinical Densitometry (ISCD) has a user-friendly precision calculator on their web site: http://iscd.org.

It is important to point out that none of the peripheral devices show changes in BMD between measurements in patients receiving antiresorptive therapy. This is not due to the precision error differences between central and peripheral devices, because the peripheral devices have precision errors that are similar to central DXA. For reasons that are unclear, none of the peripheral technologies have shown BMD changes in any of the antiresorptive clinical trials. There was, in fact, a loss of forearm BMD in patients in the anabolic trial that used PTH, which again might be an artifact of the areal DXA measurement in which the bone area is increased by teriparatide-induced subperiosteal bone apposition. One of the frustrating aspects of bone densitometry is the inability to monitor pharmacologic therapy with peripheral devices, whereas they can be used quite appropriately to assess risk. Until improved method allow peripheral devices to be used for monitoring therapy, the physician is left with three choices if he or she decides to start osteoporosis-specific therapy on the basis of the increased risk as assessed by peripheral devices:

1. Don't monitor.

2. Use axial (central DXA) as well as a baseline DXA for monitoring, because axial BMD by DXA is the preferred method for monitoring osteoporosis-specific therapies.

3. Use BCM of bone turnover to assess the bone biologic response to the antiresorptive agent. There are data to suggest that, particularly with the bisphosphonates, if there is at least a 40% drop in urinary collagen cross-link markers 1–3 months after initiating a bisphosphonate, there is a greater likelihood that the 2-year follow-up repeat DXA will increase or at least not decline.[1,18] In addition, more recent data examining the relationship between the magnitude of increase in BMD and the magnitude of decrease in BCM with the various antiresorptive agents suggest that the greater the decrease in BCM, the greater the risk reduction in vertebral and nonvertebral fractures; that the strength of this relationship was as powerful as the strength of the relationship between the changes in BMD and the risk reduction. Hence, at least for groups of patients, if a BCM declines adequately, there are some data to support that one might anticipate a fracture-reduction benefit.[19]

At this time in the clinical practice of osteoporosis, no professional scientific organization recommends substitution of BCM over DXA as a means of monitoring therapy. If anything, the two should be complimentary and used together. The advantage of the 1 to 3 month BCM assessment is that it provides earlier feedback to the patient and the clinician and that if it does decline beyond the LSC for BCM, three clinical assumptions are fair:

1. The patient is taking the drug.

2. The fastidiously absorbed oral bisphosphonates are being absorbed.

3. There is some evidence for a bone biologic effect.

Finally, it is important to address the issues of "nonresponders" as measured by BMD and the principle of regression-to-the-mean as it has been applied to clinical osteoporosis management.

It has been assumed that the "response" rate to bisphosphonates exceeds 90%. These data are all derived from clinical trials. Clinic patients differ from clinical trial patients. Clinical trial patients are carefully selected. They have no secondary diseases affecting bone nor can they be taking other drugs that might alter bone metabolism. Clinical trial patients are highly motivated and have frequent compliance (i.e., pill count) checks. None of these ideal scenarios is fullfilled by the day-in-to-day-out clinic patient. The real-world response rate to osteoporosis-specific therapies is really unknown. When patients lose BMD beyond the LSC or have no change in NTX, one must examine more closely the possible presence of secondary causes, especially asymptomatic celiac disease, a condition in which neither calcium nor oral bisphosphonates may be adequately absorbed.

The monitoring of response of the anabolic agent, intermittent injectable parathyroid hormone (teriparatide), will also use serial BMD and biomarker changes. Yet, the biomarker that will be used to monitor teriparatide will be the marker of bone formation, BSAP, or osteocalan, which increases with teriparatide bone response. Other osteoblast-derived markers may be more sensitive as indicators to monitor PTH response (P1NP, P1CP). These are, however, not commercially available. Although spine BMD by DXA does show impressive rises in BMD with teriparatide use, the wrist declines because the bone area increases. Because bone size increases with teriparatide, which will lead to the underestimation of the change in BMC, it might be valuable to monitor teriparatide with pQCT techniques, a theoretical issue.

Regression to the mean is an old statistical observation. Most recently it has been used in BMD testing to examine the change from pretreatment baseline in two pharmacologic clinical trials of PMO. The article recently published on this statistical phenomenon stated that those patients on treatment for the first 2 years of these trials who either lost or gained bone during the first year subsequently either gained or lost bone during the second year, such that when the two data points were regressed to the mean values between the two data points, there were no differences.[20] The article suggested that measuring BMD over time may not have meaning for those patients who gain BMD during the first year and lose the second year and those who lose the first year and gain the second year. One scientific flaw of these data is that they are a statistical fact that regression to the mean occurs in all biologic measurements, especially at the extremes of a distribution, such that values that are high subsequently decline and those that are low subsequently increase *because* of regression to the mean, no matter what we do—in both the treated and the control group.[21,22] In the article cited,[20] the control group data points were not shown, only the treated group's points; to know whether regression to the mean has any real meaning, the differences between the treated and nontreated groups at the regression point must be shown. Any differences between these two groups at the regression point would thus clarify whether there were differences between the treated and untreated groups. Finally, regression to the mean can never be applied to individual patients, because it is always a group phenomenon seen at the extremes of distribution.

Serial BMD and increases in BMD while on osteoporosis-specific therapies are valid surrogate markers of assessing to some degree the improvement in bone strength. BMD increases explain a significant proportion, but not all, of the fracture-risk reduction seen with antiresorptive agents. If evidence did not support this scientific fact, the FDA would not have approved the once-a-week bisphosphonate formulations that were registered on the basis of equivalent increases in BMD and reductions in BCM of bone turnover as seen with the daily formulations. If clinicians do not accept the premise that the equal BMD increases or equal reductions in BCM seen with weekly bisphosphonate formulations compared with daily dosing translate into equal fracture reduction, then clinicians should think more deeply about weekly formulations in their high-risk patients.

BMD testing has been one of the major advances in the field of osteoporosis that has allowed clinical applications in diagnosis, risk prediction, and monitoring of disease or therapy. Without BMD availability and monitoring of the pharmacologic effects, the field of the clinical management of osteoporosis would be relegated to guesswork. Yet, like all biologic measurements, BMD testing at baseline and/or longitudinally is imperfect. Only competent clinical judgment and competent clinical interpretation of bone mass measurements will allow this important quantitative technology to remain an important clinical tool. As long as clinicians assess serial BMD measurements correctly, serial BMD will remain the "gold standard" for monitoring osteoporosis therapies.

Key Points: Monitoring Osteoporosis Therapy

- ◌ Serial BMD testing and measurement of BCM of bone resorption are the best surrogate markers for monitoring the efficacy of osteoporosis-specific pharmacologic agents
- ◌ Competent serial BMD performance requires that each DXA facility know their own in vivo precision error and understand the principles of the least significant change.
- ◌ Both increases in BMD and declines in the BCM of bone resorption contribute to reduction in fracture risk with antiresorptive agents

References

1. Miller PD, Baran D, Bilezikian JP, et al: Practical clinical application of biomarkers of bone turnover. J Clin Densitom 2:323–342, 1999.
2. Nancollas GH, Mangood GH, Gaafar EM, et al: Comparative mineral binding affinities of selected bisphosphonates. Osteoporos Inter 13: S51, 2002.
3. Dunford JE, Thompson K, Coxon FP, et al: Structure-activity relationships of inhibition of farnesyl diphosphate synthetase in vitro and inhibition of bone resorption in vivo by nitrogen-containing bisphosphonates. J Pharmacol Exp Ther 2:235–242, 2001.
4. Kahn SA, Kanis JA, Vasikarin S, et al: Elimination and biochemical responses to intravenous alendronate in postmenopausal osteoporosis. J Bone Miner Res 12(10):1700–1707, 1997.
5. Nancollas GH, Mangood GH, Gaafar EM, et al: Comparative mineral binding affinities of selected bisphosphonates. Osteoporos Int 13: S51, 2002.
6. Borah B, Dufresne TE, Chimelewski PA, et al: Risedronate preserves trabecular architecture and increases bone strength in vertebrae of ovariectomized mini-pigs as measured by 3-dimensional microcomputed tomography. J Bone Miner Res 17:1139–117, 2002.
7. Wasnich RD, Miller PD: Antifracture efficacy of antiresorptive agents are related to changes in bone density. J Clin Endocrinol Metab 85:231–236, 2001.
8. Cummings SR, Karpf DB, Harris F, et al: Improvements in spine bone density and reduction in risk of vertebral fractures during treatment with antiresorptive drugs. Am J Med 114:281–289, 2002.
9. Hochburg MC, Greenspan S, Wasnich RD, et al: Changes in bone density and turnover explain the reductions in incidence of non-vertebral fractures that occur during treatment with antiresorptive agents. J Clin Endocrinol Metab 87:1586–1592, 2002.
10. Peel NFA, Eastell R: Comparison of rates of bone loss from the spine measured using two manufacturers' densitometers. J Bone Miner Res 10:1796–1801, 1995.
11. Miller PD, Bilezikian JP: Bone mineral density in asymptomatic primary hyperparathyroidism. J Bone Miner Res 17: 538–541, 2002.
12. Neer RM, Arnaud CD, Zanchetta JR, et al: Effect of parathyroid hormone (1-34) on fractures and bone mineral density in postmenopausal women with osteoporosis. N Engl J Med 344: 1434–1441, 2001.
13. Gaich GA, Zancheta JR, Bogado C, et al: Effect of terapeptide on cortical bone strength indices as assessed by peripheral quantitative computed tomography. J Bone Miner Res 16:S181, 2001.
14. Miller PD, Zapalowski C, Kulak CAM, et al: Bone densitometry: The best way to detect osteoporosis and to monitor therapy. J Clin Endocrinol Metab 84:1867–1871, 1999.
15. Bonnick SL, Johnston CC Jr, Kleerekoper M, et al: The importance of precision in bone density. J Clin Densitom 4: 105–110, 2001.
16. Gluer CC, Blake G, Lu Y, et al: Accurate assessment of precision errors: how to measure the reproducibility errors of bone densitometry. Osteoporos Int 5:262–270, 1995.
17. Lenchik L, Kiebzak G, Blunt BA: What is the role of serial BMD measurements in patients? J Clin Densitom 5 (Suppl. 1): 2002.
18. Greenspan SL, Rosen HN, Parker LA: Early changes in serum N-telopeptide and C-telopeptides cross-link collagen type I predict long-term response to alendronate therapy in post-menopausal women. J Clin Endocrinol Metab 85:3537–3540, 2000.
19. Eastell R, Barton I, Hannon RA, et al: Antifracture efficacy of risedronate: prediction by change in bone resorption markers. J Bone Miner Res 16:S163, 2001

20. Cummings SL, Palmero L, Browner L, et al: Monitoring osteoporosis therapy with bone densitometry: misleading changes and regression to the mean. JAMA 283:1318–1321, 2000.
21. Bonnick SL: Monitoring osteoporosis therapy with bone densitometry: a vital tool or regression toward mediocrity? J Clin Endocrinol Metab 10:343–345, 2000.
22. Lenchik L, Watts NM: Regression to the mean: what does it mean? J Clin Densitom 4:1–4, 2001.

Treatment after Fragility Fractures

chapter
9

Carol Zapalowski, M.D., Ph.D.

Although the intent of the prevention, detection, and treatment of osteoporosis is the prevention of the initial fragility fracture, in many cases patients are first seen after their first fracture has already occurred. The estimated lifetime risk of fragility fracture after the age of 50 is 40% for women and 13% for men.[1] When fractures occur, health is adversely affected in many ways, including reduced mobility, chronic pain, clinical depression, inability to do activities of daily living, and a significant financial burden to both the patient and society. Both hip fractures and vertebral fractures were found to be associated with an age-adjusted increased mortality of approximately 20%–25%.[2,3]

In a patient who has had a fragility fracture, bone density measurements should be performed so that the effect of therapeutic interventions can be followed over time. However, if a patient with a fragility fracture does not have osteoporosis on bone density testing, he or she is still considered to be osteoporotic by virtue of the fracture. In a patient with a fragility fracture, a full workup looking for evidence of secondary causes of osteoporosis should be initiated, independent of bone density. It is estimated that 90% of all hip and spine fractures in elderly women are attributable to osteoporosis.[4] However, it is worthwhile keeping other possible etiologies in the differential diagnosis. Malignancy should always be considered as a possible etiology in a patient with fragility fracture, especially in the setting of a normal BMD.

Despite the effects of fractures on health and the association of fragility fracture with osteoporosis, a significant proportion of patients with known osteoporotic fractures is not on specific therapeutic measures for osteoporosis. The percentage of patients on any therepy varies from study to study, ranging from 4% of patients admitted to the hospital for hip fracture in one study[5] to 32% of patients known to have vertebral compression fractures in an outpatient primary care setting.[6] Many studies show similar low percentages in this range.[7–10]

123

Prevention of Future Fragility Fractures with Pharmacologic Agents

Therapy for osteoporosis has been discussed in detail in Chapter 7. When considering therapy after a fracture, therapies that have a rapid effect should be considered. Therapy with alendronate,[11] rise-dronate,[12,13] and raloxifene[14] has been shown to decrease clinical vertebral fracture incidence within one year by greater than 40%.[15] In fact, in a post-hoc analysis, risedronate was found to decrease the risk for clinical vertebral fracture by as early as 6 months.[16] Recombinant human parathyroid hormone 1-34 was found to decrease vertebral fractures significantly by 18 months.[17] Therapy with bisphosphonates also decreases the risk for hip fracture. In studies with both risedronate[18] and alendronate,[19] there was a significant decrease in hip fracture risk at 3 years.[20] In post-hoc analyses, it seems that the bisphosphonates have a statistically significant effect on decrease in the incidence of hip fracture at 18 months.[11,21]

As discussed previously, the increased risk for subsequent fracture seen in patients with prior fragility fracture is present within the first year after the initial fracture. Therefore, it is imperative that therapy be started immediately after the diagnosis of a fragility fracture to prevent future fractures.

Vertebral Fractures

Morbidity of Vertebral Fractures

Vertebral fracture is the most common form of fragility fracture, followed by hip and wrist fractures.[22,23] Although fractures of the hip and wrist come to medical attention because of the need for therapy, there is often a failure to diagnose and treat vertebral fractures in both women and men because of a decreased level of awareness of their prevalence and, therefore, a failure of diagnosis. The prevalence of vertebral fractures increases with age from 5% at the age of 50–54 to 50% in those ages 80–84.[22,24]

It is estimated that only 30% of vertebral fractures come to clinical attention (i.e., are diagnosed).[25] Vertebral fractures can present in several ways. One-third of the time, patients have pain and are diagnosed with radiographic abnormalities consistent with the description of their back pain. There is often no history of trauma, unless it is specifically sought out. Patients who have had more than an inch of height loss should be evaluated with vertebral x-rays looking for evidence of radiographic deformities as the etiology of height loss. Although it is very common for vertebral deformities to be missed on formal readings of chest x-rays, abnormalities may be visualized on x-rays done for other reasons.[26] Whether a fracture is painful or not, a spinal deformity impacts health, daily living, and medical costs.

The most common vertebral fragility fractures occur at the midthoracic level (T7–T8) and at the thoracolumbar junction (T12–L1), but fractures can occur throughout the thoracolumbar spine[22,27,28] and even, rarely, in the cervical spine. The significance of vertebral fractures lies not only in the pain and loss of function but also in the risk of future fracture they predict. Lindsay et al[29] followed women with osteoporosis on calcium and vitamin D alone for 1 year, stratified on the basis of the number of prevalent (baseline) vertebral fractures. In women with no vertebral fractures at baseline, there was a 2% incidence of fracture within 1 year. In women with one vertebral fracture, there was a 5% incidence of new vertebral fractures in the next year, and in women with more than two vertebral fractures, there was a 13% incidence of new vertebral fractures in the following year. This indicates that previous vertebral fracture is important in predicting future fracture. In addition, women who had an incident vertebral fracture during the study were followed for another year and found to have a 19% incidence of fracture within 1 year. The increased fracture risk in the period immediately after a fracture validates the urgency of identification and intervention in patients with a prior fragility fracture.

Acute, severe back pain at the level of the vertebral fracture usually lasts 6 to 12 weeks. However, approximately three-fourths of clinically evident vertebral fractures will subsequently cause chronic pain because of a multitude of reasons, including vertebral deformity, paraspinous muscle spasm, degenerative arthritis, and changes in spinal alignment.[30,31] There is an increased 5-year mortality rate in women who have had vertebral fractures. The relative risk for survival is 80% at 5 years in women of comparable ages.[32,33] Decreased mobility and fear of falling also adversely affect quality of life after vertebral fracture. It is estimated that there is a 9% decrease in pulmonary vital capacity with each vertebral fracture, leading to impaired pulmonary function,[34] which worsens with each subsequent fracture.

Evaluation

Once a fragility fracture has been discovered, a patient should be evaluated for secondary causes of osteoporosis (see Chapter 5 for a full discussion of secondary causes). Bone density measurements should be done on all patients with a fragility fracture to give the clinician baseline BMD values in order to follow his or her therapeutic interventions over time.

Treatment of Pain

Treatment should focus not only on decreasing pain and increasing function but also on preventing future fractures and progressive disability. It is important to remember nonpharmacologic modalities as adjuncts to pharmacotherapy for pain management.[35] Local heat, cold, rest, transcutaneous electrical nerve stimulation (TENS) units, massage therapy, walking aids, and back braces have not been studied specifically for osteoporotic vertebral fracture and have had varying success rates in the treatment of back pain of other etiologies. Exercise programs have been shown to decrease the use of analgesics and improve function after vertebral fracture.[36] Balance training programs such as Tai Chi have achieved a decrease in the risk of falls.[37]

The pharmacotherapy for acute pain from vertebral fractures includes analgesics such as acetaminophen and nonsteroidal antiinflammatory drugs, if there is no medical contraindication. Narcotic analgesics should be used with caution because of the risk of delirium and gait instability in the patient already at high risk for falls and, thereby, subsequent fragility fractures. In patients with pain from acute vertebral fractures, calcitonin by subcutaneous or nasal daily administration was found to have an analgesic effect, at least in some studies.[38,39] Because it is a medication with very few side effects, it is certainly reasonable to consider nasal calcitonin in conjunction with other analgesics. The analgesic effect of calcitonin should be seen within 2 weeks. Usually calcitonin is used short term (i.e., for approximately 6 months in the setting of an acute fracture), because there are no substantial data for chronic pain relief for vertebral fractures. There is less fracture prevention data with calcitonin than other agents, as discussed in Chapter 6. Therefore, when calcitonin is used as an analgesic, it should be used in conjunction with another agent for treatment of osteoporosis.

Vertebroplasty and Kyphoplasty

Kyphoplasty and vertebroplasty have a role in the treatment of painful osteoporotic vertebral compression fractures that do not respond to conventional treatments. Substantial pain relief was reported in most patients treated with both vertebroplasty and kyphoplasty.[40–47] Although pain relief seems to be equivalent with both vertebroplasty and kyphoplasty, kyphoplasty offers the advantage of improving spinal alignment and partially restoring vertebral height. There have been no prospective, randomized, controlled studies comparing vertebroplasty or kyphoplasty with medical management to determine the relative safety and efficacy, and, therefore, clinical indications for vertebroplasty and kyphoplasty must still be clarified.

Kyphoplasty and vertebroplasty can be considered for patients with a painful osteoporotic compression fracture in the thoracic or lumbar vertebrae. Patients are candidates for the procedure if they have had short-term medical therapy for pain control fail or have evidence of progressive kyphosis. Postoperatively, the patient is usually observed for several hours in the recovery room. Pain relief is frequently immediate. Contraindications include acute traumatic fractures, an age of <40 years, burst fractures with middle column disruption, solid metastatic tumors, bleeding disorders, and technically difficult situations such as vertebra plana.[46]

Vertebroplasty involves the percutaneous injection of methylmethacrylate into a fractured vertebral body under fluoroscopic guidance. The purpose of vertebroplasty is for control of pain after acute vertebral fracture. The procedure is usually performed under local or general anesthesia by an interventional radiologist, orthopedist, or anesthesiologist. The procedure was first developed in the 1980s for treatment of pathologic fractures. The methylmethacrylate is injected under pressure. This procedure is done mainly for pain control and has not been shown to correct the compression deformity of the fractured vertebra. It is postulated that pain relief comes from stabilizing the fractured vertebral body with bone cement. The major potential risk of vertebroplasty is extravasation of methylmethacrylate into the epidural space. Cement leakages have been reported in 30%–67% of patients undergoing vertebroplasty, but fewer than 10% had epidural leakage and only 4% reported radiculopathy.[48] Case series of patients treated with vertebral fractures with vertebroplasty reported improvement of pain in 70%–90% of patients.[41]

Kyphoplasty involves the percutaneous insertion of a balloon into a collapsed vertebral body, followed by inflation of the balloon with radiographic contrast. This reexpands the vertebral body. With kyphoplasty, an intravertebral cavity surrounded by compacted cancellous bone is created by balloon inflation. This allows for low-pressure filling of the cavity with methylmethacrylate. This procedure restores vertebral height, decreases deformity, and reduces pain with a lower risk of cement extravasation than vertebroplasty.[49] Kyphoplasty is most successful at restoring vertebral height when performed within 3 months of a fracture.

The complication rate of kyphoplasty seems to be less than that of vertebroplasty. Possible long-term complications of both procedures include local acceleration of bone resorption and increased risk of fracture in adjacent vertebrae.[50] In some patients, new compression fractures have been observed in adjacent levels after the procedure.[51] Although the incident fractures observed after kyphoplasty could be an expression of the natural course of the disease, they also may be the result of rigid reinforcement in the adjacent vertebrae. The presence of a rigid cement augmentation may facilitate the subsequent collapse of adjacent vertebrae.[50] Last, serious neurologic complications such as radiculopathy and spinal cord compression have been anecdotally reported with these procedures. These complications seem to be uncommon by reports in the literature, but the rate and significance of complications have yet to be clarified and reported for each procedure, and carefully controlled outcome studies are needed.

Hip Fracture

Hip fracture is a considerable worry for most elderly women. One survey of women 75 years of age and older showed that 80% would rather be dead than experience the loss of independence that results from a hip fracture and subsequent admission to a nursing home.[52] The risk for hip fracture is increased in patients with prior hip fracture and in patients with prior vertebral fracture.[53] After hip fracture, people experience a significant decrease in health-related quality of life.[54] One year after hip fracture, 40% of patients are still unable to walk independently, 60% have difficulty with at least one essential activity of daily living, and 80% are restricted in other activities, such as driving and grocery shopping. Moreover, 27% of these patients enter a nursing home for the first time.[3] There is a 20%–25% increase in mortality rate seen in the first year after hip fracture, and among survivors, the number requiring admission to a long-term facility is double that of age- and gender-matched controls.[55]

As discussed previously for vertebral fractures, any person with fragility fracture, in this case hip fracture, deserves a workup for secondary causes of osteoporosis and a baseline bone density evaluation. In addition, therapy for osteoporosis should be started as soon as the workup is complete and the most appropriate medication identified.

Most immediate post–hip fracture care happens through orthopedics, (i.e., with the surgeons who do the surgical intervention). It is important to minimize the use of sedating medications to prevent future fractures caused by drowsiness, confusion, and increased risk for fall. When possible, get patients up and walking as soon as possible. Immobility and lack of activity result in decreased bone mass. Note that walking is associated with a decreased risk for hip fracture.[56–59] All patients who are candidates should be referred for physical therapy as soon as possible to facilitate the return to the highest activity level possible. In addition, patients are often receiving venous thromboembolism prophylaxis medications, which can result in bone loss as well.[60–62]

Many factors contribute to increased bone loss in the perioperative period. These patients are already at increased fracture risk solely because of their history of fragility fracture. Therefore, it is imperative to expedite the evaluation and treatment of the underlying osteoporosis. Excellent therapeutic interventions that can avoid subsequent vertebral and hip fractures are readily available and should be started as quickly as possible to improve the quality of life of patients with osteoporosis and fragility fracture.

Key Points: Treatment after Fragility Fractures

- Fragility fractures have a high morbidity and mortality.
- Fragility fractures predict future fragility fractures.
- Evaluation and treatment should be started immediately after recognition of a fragility fracture.
- Kyphoplasty and vertebroplasty can be considered for painful osteoporotic compression fractures in the thoracic and lumbar vertebrae, although there have been no prospective randomized controlled studies comparing these procedures with medical management of vertebral fractures.
- Immobility and lack of activity result in loss of bone mass. All patients should be referred for physical therapy as soon as possible after hip and spine fractures.

References

1. Melton LJ III, Lane A, Cooper C, et al: Prevalence and incidence of vertebral deformities. Osteoporos Int 3:113–119, 1993.
2. Cooper C, Atkinson EJ, Jacobsen SJ, et al: Population-based study of survival after osteoporotic fractures. Am J Epidemiol 137:1001–1005, 1993.
3. Cooper C: The crippling consequences of fractures and their impact on quality of life. Am J Med 103:12S–7S, 1997.
4. Melton LJ, Thamer M, Ray NF, et al: Fractures attributable to osteoporosis: report from the National Osteoporosis Foundation. J Bone Miner Res 12:16–23, 1997.
5. Malik R: Prevalence of osteoporosis treatment in hip fracture patients. J Am Geriatr Soc 51(Suppl 4):S118, 2003.
6. Neuner JM, Zimmer JK, Hamel MB: Diagnosis and treatment of osteoporosis in patients with vertebral compression fractures. J Am Geriatr Soc 51(4):483–491, 2003.
7. Kamel HK, Hussain MS, Tariq S, et al: Failure to diagnose and treat osteoporosis in elderly patients hospitalized with hip fracture. Am J Med 109:326–328, 2000.

8. Khan S, De Geus C, Holroyd B, et al: Osteoporosis follow-up after wrist fractures following minor trauma. Arch Intern Med 161:1309–1312, 2001.

9. Bellantonio S, Fortinsky R: How well are community-living women treated for osteoporosis after hip fracture? J Am Geriatr Soc 49:1197–1204, 2001.

10. Freedman K, Kaplan F, Bilker W, et al: Treatment of osteoporosis: Are physicians missing an opportunity? J Bone Joint Surg Am 82:1063–1070, 2000.

11. Black DM, Thompson DE, Bauer DC, et al.: Fracture risk reduction with alendronate in women with osteoporosis: the Fracture Intervention Trial. FIT Research Group. J Clin Endocrinol Metab 85:4118–4124, 2000.

12. Harris ST, Watts NB, Genant HK, et al: Effects of risedronate treatment on vertebral and nonvertebral fractures in women with postmenopausal osteoporosis: a randomized controlled trial. Vertebral Efficacy With Risedronate Therapy (VERT) Study Group. JAMA 282:1344–352, 1999.

13. Reginster J, Minne HW, Sorensen OH, et al: Randomized trial of the effects of risedronate on vertebral fractures in women with established postmenopausal osteoporosis. Vertebral Efficacy with Risedronate Therapy (VERT) Study Group. Osteoporos Int 11:83–91, 2000.

14. Maricic M, Adachi JD, Sarkar S, et al: Early effects of raloxifene on clinical vertebral fractures at 12 months in postmenopausal women with osteoporosis. Arch Intern Med 162:1140–1143, 2002.

15. Miller P: Analysis of 1-year vertebral fracture risk reduction data in treatments for osteoporosis. South Med J 96(5):478–485, 2003.

16. Watts NB, Adami S, Chesnut CH: Risedronate reduces the risk of clinical vertebral fractures in just 6 months. J Bone Miner Res 16(1):S407, 2001.

17. Neer RM, Arnaud CD, Zanchetta JR, et al: Effect of parathyroid hormone (1-34) on fractures and bone mineral density in postmenopausal women with osteoporosis. N Engl J Med 344:1434–1441, 2001.

18. McClung MR, Geusens P, Miller PD, et al: Effect of risedronate on the risk of hip fracture in elderly women. Hip Intervention Program Study Group. N Engl J Med 344:333–40, 2001.

19. Black DM, Cummings SR, Karpf DB, et al: Randomized trial of effect of alendronate on risk of fracture in women with existing vertebral fractures. Fracture Intervention Trial Research Group. Lancet 348:1535–1541, 1996.

20. Cranney A, Tugwell P, Zytaruk N, et al: The Osteoporosis Methodology Group and The Osteoporosis Research Advisory Group: Meta-analyses of therapies for postmenopausal osteoporosis. VI. Meta-analysis of calcitonin for the treatment of postmenopausal osteoporosis. Endocr Rev 23(4):540–551, 2002.

21. Chesnut C, Bolognese M, Barton I, et al: The rapid effect of risedronate on the risk of clinical vertebral fractures and non-vertebral fractures in women with postmenopausal osteoporosis, abstract at International Society of Clinical Densitometry Meeting, Los Angeles, February 2003.

22. Genant HK, Cooper C, Poor G, et al: Interim report and recommendations of the World Health Organization task-force for osteoporosis. Osteoporos Int 10:259–264, 1999.

23. Osteoporosis: review of the evidence for the prevention, diagnosis and treatment and cost-effectiveness analyses. Osteoporos Int 8(4):S1–S80, 1998.

24. Melton LJ III, Kan SH, Frye MA, et al: Epidemiology of vertebral fractures in women. Am J Epidemiol 129:1000–1011, 1989.

25. Cooper C, Melton LJ III.: Vertebral fractures: how large is the silent epidemic? BMJ 304:793–794, 1992.

26. Gehlbach SH, Bigelow C, Heimisdottir M, et al: Recognition of vertebral fracture in a clinical setting. Osteoporos Int 11(7):577–582, 2000.

27. Cooper C, Atkinson EJ, O'Fallon WM, et al: Incidence of clinically diagnosed verte-bral fractures: a population-based study in Rochester, Minnesota, 1985–1989. J Bone Miner Res 7:221–227, 1992.

28. Melton LJ III, Lane A, Cooper C, et al: Prevalence and incidence of vertebral defor-mities. Osteoporos Int 3:113–119, 1993.

29. Lindsay R, Silverman SL, Cooper C, et al: Risk of new vertebral fracture in the year following a fracture. JAMA 285:320–323, 2001.

30. Cook DJ, Guyatt GH, Adachi JD, et al: Quality of life issues in women with vertebral fractures due to osteoporosis. Arthritis Rheum 36:750–756, 1993.

31. Lyles KW, Gold DT, Shipp KM, et al: Association of osteoporotic vertebral fractures with impaired functional status. Am J Med 94:595–601, 1993.

32. Kado DM, Browner WS, Palermo L, et al: Vertebral fractures and mortality in older women: a prospective study. Study of Osteoporotic Fractures Research Group. Arch Intern Med 159:1215–1220, 1999.

33. Cooper C, Atkinson EJ, Jacobsen SJ, et al: Population-based study of survival after osteoporotic fractures. Am J Epidemiol 137:1001–1005, 1993.

34. Leech JA, Dulberg C, Kellie S, et al: Relationship of lung function to severity of osteo-porosis in women. Am Rev Respir Dis 141:68–71, 1990.

35. Tamayo-Orozco J, Arzac-Palumbo P, Peon-Vidales H, et al: Vertebral fractures associ-ated with osteoporosis: patient management. Am J Med 103(2A):44S–48S, 1997.

36. Malmros B, Mortensen L, Jensen MB, et al: Positive effect of physiotherapy on chronic pain and performance in osteoporosis. Osteoporos Int 8:215–221, 1998.

37. Wolf SL, Barnhart HX, Kutner NG: Reducing fragility and falls in older persons: an investigation of tai chi and computerized balance training. Atlanta FICSIT Group. Fragility and Injuries: Cooperative Studies of Intervention Techniques. J Am Geriatr Soc 44:599–600, 1996.

38. Gennari C: Analgesic effect of calcitonin in osteoporosis. Bone 30(5):67S–70S, 2002.

39. Lyritis GP, Trovas G: Analgesic effects of calcitonin. Bone 30(5):71S–74S, 2002.

40. Lieberman IH, Dudeney S, Reinhardt MK, et al: Initial outcome and efficacy of kyphoplasty in the treatment of painful osteoporotic vertebral compression fractures. Spine 26:1631–1638, 2001.

41. Watts NB, Harris ST, Genant HK: Treatment of painful osteoporotic vertebral fractures with percutaneous vertebroplasty or kyphoplasty. Osteoporos Int 12:429–437, 2001.

42. Garfin SR, Yuan H, Deiley MA: New technology in spine: kyphoplasty and vertebroplasty for the treatment of painful body compression fractures. Spine 26:1511–1575, 2001.

43. Garfin SR: A retrospective review of early outcomes of balloon kyphoplasty. Proceedings of the 16th Annual Meeting of the North American Spine Society, Seattle, Washington, 2001.

44. Papaioannou A, Watts NB, Kendler DL, et al: Diagnosis and management of vertebral fractures in elderly adults. Am J Med 113:220–228, 2002.

45. Lin JT, Lane JM: Nonmedical management of osteoporosis. Curr Opin Rheumatol 14:441–446, 2002.

46. Hanley E, Green NE, Spengler DM: Less invasive procedures in spine surgery. J Bone Joint Surg Ame 85A(5):956–961, 2003.

47. Truumees E: The roles of vertebroplasty and kyphoplasty as parts of a treatment strategy for osteoporotic vertebral compression fractures. Curr Opin Orthop 13(3):193–199, 2002.

48. Chiras J: Percutaneous vertebral surgery: techniques and indications. J Neuroradiol 24:45–52, 1997.

49. Phillips FM, Todd-Wetzel F, Lieberman I, et al: An in vivo comparison of the poten-tial for extravertebral cement leak after vertebroplasty and kyphoplasty. Spine 27:2173–2178, 2002.

50. Berlemann U, Ferguson SJ, Nolte LP, et al: Adjacent vertebral failure after vertebroplasty. A biomechanical investigation. J Bone Joint Surg Br 84(5):748–752, 2002.
51. Grados F, Depriester C, Cayrolle G, et al: Long-term observations of vertebral osteoporotic fractures treated by percutaneous vertebroplasty. Rheumatology 39:1410–1414, 2000.
52. Salkeld G, Cameron ID, Cumming RG, et al: Quality of life related to fear of falling and hip fracture in older women: a time trade off study. BMJ 320:341–346, 2000.
53. Black DM, Arden NK, Palermo L, et al: Prevalent vertebral deformities predict hip fractures and new vertebral deformities but not wrist fractures. Study of Osteoporotic Fractures Research Group. J Bone Miner Res 14:821–828, 1999.
54. Randell AG, Nguyen TV, Bhalerao N, et al: Deterioration in quality of life following hip fracture: a prospective study. Osteoporos Int 11:460–466, 2000.
55. Jalovaara P, Virkkunen H: Quality of life after primary hemiarthroplasty for femoral neck fracture. 6-year follow-up of 185 patients. Acta Orthop Scand 62:208–1217, 1991.
56. Feskanich D, Willett W, Colditz G: Walking and leisure-time activity and risk of hip fracture in postmenopausal women. JAMA 288(18):2300–2306, 2002.
57. Paganini-Hill A, Chao A, Ross RK, et al: Exercise and other factors in the prevention of hip fracture: the Leisure World study. Epidemiology 2(1):16–25, 1991.
58. Gregg EW, Cauley JA, Seeley DG, et al: Physical activity and osteoporotic fracture risk in older women. Study of Osteoporotic Fractures Research Group. Ann Intern Med 129(2):81–88, 1998.
59. Hoidrup S, Sorensen TIA, Stroger U, et al: Leisure-time physical activity levels and changes in relation to risk of hip fracture in men and women. Am J Epidemiol 154(1):60–68, 2001.
60. Sullivan SD, Kahn SR, Davidson BL, et al: Measuring the outcomes and pharmacoeconomic consequences of venous thromboembolism prophylaxis in major orthopaedic surgery. Pharmacoeconomics 21(7):477–496, 2003.
61. Nelson-Piercy C: Hazards of heparin: allergy, heparin-induced thrombocytopenia and osteoporosis. Baillieres Clin Obstet Gynaecol 11:489–509, 1997.
62. Jamal SA, Browner WS, Bauer DC, et al: Warfarin use and risk for osteoporosis in elderly women. Study of Osteoporotic Fractures Research Group. Ann Intern Med 128(10):829–832, 1998.

Glucocorticoid-induced Osteoporosis

chapter
10

Michael T. McDermott, M.D.

Harvey Cushing described Cushing's syndrome in 1932.[1] In his initial description of this disease, he noted that "the greatly compressed bodies of the vertebra . . . were so soft that they could easily be cut with a knife." When glucocorticoids were first used for the treatment of chronic inflammatory disorders in the 1950s, it soon became apparent that these bone changes occurred with exogenous steroid administration as well.[2] Glucocorticoid-induced osteoporosis is presently the most common cause of drug-induced osteoporosis. Significant bone loss and skeletal fractures may occur within 6 months of starting glucocorticoid therapy, and up to 50% of individuals on chronic glucocorticoid treatment will develop an osteoporotic fracture.[3]

The amount of bone loss that occurs and the magnitude of the fracture risk are clearly related to both the dose and the duration of glucocorticoid therapy. Supraphysiologic glucocorticoid doses ($\geq$ 7.5 mg of prednisone or equivalent) are associated with the greatest risk. However, a large retrospective cohort study involving 244,235 individuals who had received glucocorticoid therapy showed a significantly increased fracture risk even in those whose median prednisolone doses had been as low as 2.5 mg/day[4] (Fig. 10-1). Bone loss has also been reported in patients receiving replacement glucocorticoid therapy for primary adrenal insufficiency,[5] indicating that individuals on any dose of oral glucocorticoid therapy may be at risk for osteoporosis. Decreased BMD and an increased risk of fragility fractures have even been demonstrated in patients using only inhaled glucocorticoids.[6–9]

The pathogenesis of glucocorticoid-induced osteoporosis is still not entirely clear, but there has been significant recent progress in explaining its mechanisms.[10–14] Glucocorticoids are known to adversely affect both phases of bone remodeling, simultaneously decreasing bone formation and increasing bone resorption (Fig. 10-2). Glucocorticoids

133

Figure 10-1. Glucocorticoid therapy increases the risk of skeletal fractures. In this retrospective cohort study of 244,235 subjects who had received treatment with glucocorticoids, the risk of vertebral fractures was increased by 55% (adjusted relative rate, 1.55; 95% CI, 1.20–2.01) in those whose mean daily prednisolone dose was < 2.5 mg/day, by 159% (adjusted relative rate, 2.59; 95% CI, 2.16–3.10) in those whose mean daily prednisolone dose was 2.5–7.5 mg/day, and by 418% (adjusted relative rate, 5.18; 95% CI, 4.25–6.31) in those whose mean daily prednisolone dose was > 7.5 mg/day. (Adapted from Van Staa TP, et al: Use of oral corticosteroids and risk of fractures). J Bone Miner Res 15:993–1000, 2000.

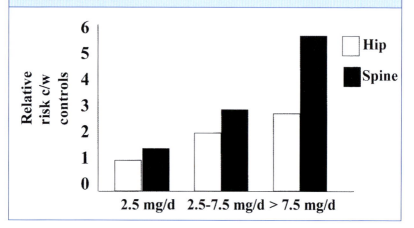

directly impair bone formation by promoting cell death (apoptosis) of existing osteoblasts and by reducing the development of new osteoblasts, most likely through inhibitory effects on local growth factors such as IGF-1. At the same time, they increase bone resorption through several indirect mechanisms, which include decreasing the production of sex steroids (estrogen and testosterone) and reducing the synthesis of osteoprotegerin, an endogenous inhibitor of osteoclastic bone resorption. These dual effects explain why such rapid bone loss can occur after the initiation of glucocorticoid therapy.

All patients taking glucocorticoid therapy should therefore be considered at risk for the development of osteoporosis and should be monitored carefully for this complication. Our recommendations for BMD testing in glucocorticoid-treated patients are shown in Table 10-1. The ideal BMD criteria for the diagnosis of glucocorticoid-induced osteoporosis are still being debated, but the best existing evidence suggests that the fracture risk per BMD decrement does not differ between glucocorticoid-treated patients and patients with primary osteoporosis.[15] Accordingly, at present, the same BMD criteria should be used to diagnose osteoporosis in these patients as in patients who are not taking glu-

> **Figure 10-2.** **Pathophysiology of glucocorticoid-induced osteoporosis.** Glucocorticoids suppress osteoblastic bone formation by promoting apoptosis of existing osteoblasts and by decreasing recruitment of new osteoblasts, at least partly through inhibitory effects on local growth factors, such as IGF-I. Glucocorticoids also indirectly increase osteoclastic bone resorption by several mechanisms, including lowering of gonadal steroid (estrogen, testosterone) secretion and reduced production of osteoprotegerin, an endogenous inhibitor of osteoclastic function. The combined effects of suppressed bone formation and enhanced bone resorption result in the rapid bone loss that is characteristic of glucocorticoid-induced osteoporosis.

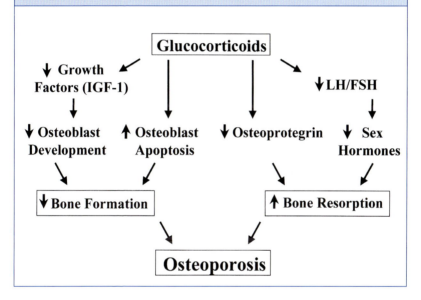

cocorticoids. However, because of the rapidity of bone loss in this condition, active treatment should be considered at an earlier stage (T score < −1.0).

Our recommendations for nonpharmacologic prevention and treatment measures for glucocorticoid-induced osteoporosis are also shown in Table 10-1. All glucocorticoid-treated patients should be advised to consume adequate calcium (1500 mg/day; combination of dietary intake plus supplements) and vitamin D (800 units/day), to exercise regularly (aerobic and resistance), to stop smoking, and to limit or discontinue alcohol consumption.

The bisphosphonates, a class of potent antiresorptive agents, have been demonstrated in numerous trials to effectively counteract the catabolic effects of glucocorticoid therapy.[16–22] A 2002 comprehensive meta-regression analysis[23] of all adequately designed and reported clinical trials determined that bisphosphonates produced a mean spine

Table 10-1. Recommendations for the Management of Glucocorticoid-treated Patients
I. Bone mineral density (BMD) testing

A. Patients: Starting glucocorticoid therapy (prednisone dose ≥ 5 mg/day or equivalent) with planned duration of treatment ≥ 3 months or on existing treatment for ≥ 3 months
B. Recommendations:
  • BMD of spine and/or hip at initiation of glucocorticoid therapy or as soon as possible thereafter
  • Repeat BMD every 6–12 months as long as glucocorticoid therapy is continued

II. Nonpharmacologic prevention and treatment measures

A. Patients: All glucocorticoid-treated patients
B. Recommendations:
  • Calcium intake: 1500 mg/day
  • Vitamin D intake: 800 IU/day
  • Exercise: aerobic and resistance
  • Habit alteration: stop smoking, limit or stop alcohol

III. Pharmacologic prevention and treatment measures

A. Patients
  • Postmenopausal women (all)
  • Men and premenopausal women with T score < -1.0
B. Recommendations:
  • Bisphosphonates: currently first line
    Oral (alendronate, risedronate, etidronate)
    Intravenous (pamidronate)
  • Teriparatide: consider when,
    Very low BMD
    Existing fragility fractures
    Inadequate response to bisphosphonates
  • Calcitonin: consider when intolerance or contraindication to bisphosphonate
  • Gonadal steroids: in combination with above or alone
    Postmenopausal women
    Hypogonadal men (low serum testosterone)
  • Thiazide diuretics:
    If urine calcium > 300 mg/day in men
    If urine calcium > 250 mg/day in women

BMD increment of 4.6%, whereas the reported mean increase was 2.3% for calcitonin and 2.9% for sodium fluoride (Fig. 10-3). Sex steroid replacement also showed beneficial effects on BMD in glucocorticoid-treated postmenopausal women[24] and men with low serum testosterone levels.[25] Teriparatide, a newly released anabolic parathyroid hormone fragment (1-34 PTH), has been reported to increase spine BMD by an impressive 9.8% (DXA) when given to glucocorticoid-

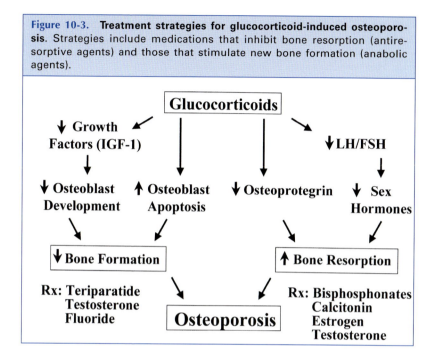

Figure 10-3. **Treatment strategies for glucocorticoid-induced osteoporosis.** Strategies include medications that inhibit bone resorption (antiresorptive agents) and those that stimulate new bone formation (anabolic agents).

treated postmenopausal women who were also on hormone replacement therapy[26,27] (Fig. 10-4). The only agents for which fracture data are available, however, are the oral bisphosphonates, which have been reported to decrease the incidence of vertebral fractures by 40–70%[18–20] (Fig. 10-5).

On the basis of the previous BMD and fracture data, oral bisphosphonates (alendronate [Fosamax], risedronate [Actonel], etidronate [Didronel]) are currently considered the agents of choice for the pharmacologic prevention and treatment of glucocorticoid-induced osteoporosis.[28,29] Intravenous pamidronate [Aredia] (or perhaps zoledronate [Zometa]), once further studies are done) may be useful as an alternative approach for patients who do not tolerate or absorb oral bisphosphonates. Calcitonin nasal spray (Miacalcin) should be considered for patients in whom the bisphosphonates are contraindicated. Estrogen replacement in postmenopausal women (after consideration of the issues discussed in Chapter 7) and testosterone replacement in hypogonadal men may also be used adjunctively but should not, in most cases, be substituted for bisphosphonate therapy. The role of teriparatide (Forteo) is still being defined in this disorder. However, in view of the profound reductions in bone formation caused by glucocorticoid therapy, this medication may prove to be a highly effective agent, alone or

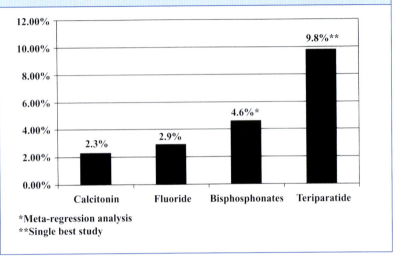

Figure 10-4. Antiresorptive and anabolic agents increase bone mass in glucocorticoid-induced osteoporosis. Illustrated are the increases in spine bone mineral density (BMD) reported in a meta-regression analysis (*) and a single study (**) examining the effects of various medications in patients with this disorder. (Adapted from Amin S, et al: The comparative efficacy of drug therapies used for the management of corticosteroid-induced osteoporosis a meta-regression. J Bone Min Res 17:1512–1526, 2000; and Lane NE, et al: Parathyroid hormone treatment can reverse corticosteroid-induced osteoporosis, results of a randomized controlled clinical trial. J Clin Invest 102: 1627–1633, 1998.)

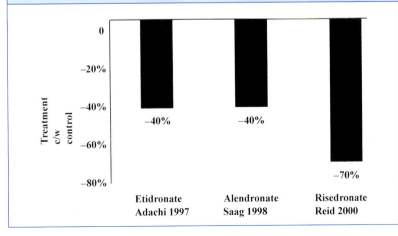

Figure 10-5. Bisphosphonates reduce vertebral fractures in glucocorticoid-induced osteoporosis. Illustrated are the results of three studies that have examined vertebral fracture occurrence in patients with glucocorticoid-induced osteoporosis treated with etidronate, alendronate, or risedronate.

in combination with antiresorptive drugs. It may be particularly useful for patients on high glucocorticoid doses or prolonged courses of glucocorticoid therapy and for those with very low BMD or who fail to respond to antiresorptive monotherapy. Additional studies with more extensive prospective fracture-reduction data using single agents and combination therapy will be necessary before the ideal therapeutic regimen for this condition can be defined. In the absence of such information, our current recommendations for pharmacologic management of glucocorticoid-induced osteoporosis are outlined in Table 10–1.

Key Points: Glucocorticoid-induced Osteoporosis

- Glucocorticoid-induced osteoporosis is the most common type of drug-induced osteoporosis.
- High doses and prolonged use of glucocorticoids produce greater risk, but all doses of oral glucocorticoids and even inhaled steroids seem to increase the risk of osteoporotic fractures.
- The pathophysiology of glucocorticoid-induced osteoporosis involves both suppressed bone formation and enhanced bone resorption, accounting for the rapid bone loss often seen in glucocorticoid-treated patients.
- BMD testing is recommended before initiation of glucocorticoid therapy in patients who will receive ≥ 5 mg/day of prednisone (or equivalent) for ≥ 3 months duration and every 6–12 months thereafter, as long as glucocorticoid therapy is continued.
- Treatment is recommended for all postmenopausal women regardless of initial BMD and for men or premenopausal women with a BMD T score < −1.0 who are being treated or will be treated with ≥ 5 mg/day of prednisone (or equivalent) for ≥ 3 months.
- Both antiresorptive and anabolic agents improve BMD in patients with glucocorticoid-induced osteoporosis.
- Bisphosphonates have been shown to reduce fragility-fracture risk in patients with glucocorticoid-induced osteoporosis.

References

1. Cushing H: The basophil adenomas of the pituitary body and their clinical manifestations (pituitary basophilism). Bull Johns Hopkins Hosp 50:137–195, 1932.
2. Curtiss PH, Clark WS, Herndon CH: Vertebral fractures resulting from prolonged cortisone and corticotrophin therapy. JAMA 156:467–9, 1954.
3. Adinoff AD, Hollister JR: Steroid-induced fractures and bone loss in patients with asthma. N Engl J Med 309:265–268, 1983.

4. Van Staa TP, Leufkens HGM, Abenhaim L, et al: Use of oral corticosteroids and risk of fractures. J Bone Miner Res 15:993–1000, 2000.

5. Zelissen PMJ, Croughs RJM, van Rijk PP, et al: Effect of glucocorticoid replacement therapy on bone mineral density in patients with Addison disease. Ann Intern Med 120:207–210, 1994.

6. Ip M, Lam K, Yam L, et al: Decreased bone mineral density in premenopausal asthma patients receiving long-term inhaled steroids. Chest 105:1722–27, 1994.

7. Ebeling PR, Erbas B, Hopper JL, et al: Bone mineral density and bone turnover in asthmatics treated with long-term inhaled or oral glucocorticoids. J Bone Miner Res 13:1283–1289, 1998.

8. Isreal E, Banerjee TR, Fitzmaurice GM, et al: Effects of inhaled glucocorticoids on bone density in premenopausal women. N Engl J Med 345:941–947, 2001.

9. Van Staa, TP, Leufkens HGM, Cooper C: Use of inhaled corticosteroids and risk of fractures. J Bone Miner Res 16:581–588, 2001.

10. Lukert BP, Raisz LG: Glucocorticoid-induced osteoporosis: pathogenesis and management. Ann Intern Med 112:352–364, 1990.

11. Ishida Y, Heersche JNM: Glucocorticoid-induced osteoporosis: both in vivo and in vitro concentrations of glucocorticoids higher than physiological levels attenuate osteoblast differentiation. J Bone Miner Res 12:1822–1826, 1998.

12. Manolagas SC, Weinstein RS: New developments in the pathogenesis and treatment of steroid-induced osteoporosis. J Bone Miner Res 14:1061–1066, 1999.

13. Canalis E: Glucocorticoid–induced osteoporosis. Curr Opin Endocrinol Diabetes 7:320–324, 2000.

14. Rubin MR, Bilezikian JP: The role of parathyroid hormone in the pathogenesis of glucocorticoid-induced osteoporosis: a re-examination of the evidence. J Clin Endocrinol Metab 87:4033–4041, 2002.

15. Selby PL, Halsey JP, Adams KRH, et al: Corticosteroids do not alter the threshold for vertebral fracture. J Bone Miner Res 15:952–956, 2000.

16. Roux C, Oriente P, Laan R, et al: Randomized trial of effect of cyclical etidronate in the prevention of corticosteroid-induced bone loss. Ciblos study group. J Clin Endocrinol Metab 83:1128–1133, 1998.

17. Geusens P, Dequeker J, Vanhoof J, et al: Cyclical etidronate increases bone density in the spine and hip of postmenopausal women receiving long term corticosteroid treatment. A double blind, randomized placebo controlled study. Ann Rheum Dis 57:724–727, 1998.

18. Adachi JD, Bensen WG, Brown J, et al: Intermittent etidronate therapy to prevent corticosteroid-induced osteoporosis. N Engl J Med 337:382–387, 1997.

19. Saag KG, Emkey R, Schnitzer TJ, et al: Alendronate for the prevention and treatment of glucocorticoid-induced osteoporosis. N Engl J Med 339:292–299, 1998.

20. Reid DM, Hughes RA, Laan RF, et al: Efficacy and safety of daily risedronate in the treatment of corticosteroid-induced osteoporosis in men and women: a randomized trial. European corticosteroid-induced osteoporosis treatment study. J Bone Miner Res 15:1006–1103, 2000.

21. Cohen S, Levy RM, Keller M, et al: Risedronate therapy prevents corticosteroid-induced bone loss: a twelve-month, multi-center, randomized, double-blind, placebo-controlled, parallel-group study. Arthritis Rheum 42:2309–2318, 1999.

22. Boutsen Y, Jamart J, Esselinckx W, et al: Primary prevention of glucocorticoid-induced osteoporosis with intravenous pamidronate and calcium: a prospective controlled 1-year study comparing a single infusion, an infusion given once every 3 months, and calcium alone. J Bone Miner Res 16(1):104–112, 2001.

23. Amin S, LaValley MP, Simms RW, et al: The comparative efficacy of drug therapies used for the management of corticosteroid-induced osteoporosis: a meta-regression. J Bone Miner Res 17:1512–1526, 2002.
24. Hall GM, Daniels M, Doyle DV, et al: Effect of hormone replacement therapy on bone mass in rheumatoid arthritis patients treated with and without steroids. Arthritis Rheum 37:1499–1505, 1994.
25. Reid IR, Wattie DJ, Evans MC, et al: Testosterone therapy in glucocorticoid-treated men. Arch Intern Med 156:1173–1177, 1996.
26. Lane NE, Sanchez S, Modin GW, et al: Parathyroid hormone treatment can reverse corticosteroid-induced osteoporosis. Results of a randomized controlled clinical trial. J Clin Invest 102:1627–1633, 1998.
27. Lane NE, Sanchez S, Modin GW, et al: Bone mass continues to increase at the hip after parathyroid hormone treatment is discontinued in glucocorticoid-induced osteoporosis: results of a randomized controlled clinical trial. J Bone Miner Res 15:944–951, 2000.
28. Adachi JD, Olszynski WP, Hanley DA, et al: Management of corticosteroid-induced osteoporosis. Semin in Arth Rheum 29:228–251, 2000.
29. American College of Rheumatology Ad Hoc committee on Glucocorticoid-Induced Osteoporosis. Recommendations for the prevention and treatment of glucocorticoid-induced osteoporosis. 2001 update. Arth Rheum 44:1496–1503, 2001.

Osteoporosis in Men

Michael T. McDermott, MD

chapter
11

Although osteoporosis occurs much more commonly in women, it clearly constitutes a significant public health problem in men as well.[1,2] Approximately 1–2 million men in the United States have osteoporosis by bone densitometry criteria and are therefore at high risk for skeletal fractures. Worldwide, approximately 30% of hip fractures occur in men. Men have a substantially higher risk of having a hip fracture than they do of having prostate cancer and have a higher mortality rate after hip fractures than do women.[3,4] Elderly men have a 25% lifetime risk of sustaining any type of osteoporotic fracture. Although guidelines for screening and reimbursement remain contentious issues, we recommend screening for osteoporosis in men who have significant risk factors for osteoporosis and in otherwise healthy men age 75 years or older.

The greatest area of current controversy is how to make the diagnosis of osteoporosis in men. Certainly, the presence of a fragility fracture (low/no trauma fracture of a vertebra, hip, or wrist) establishes the diagnosis, provided no other metabolic bone disease can be identified as the culprit. However, bone densitometry criteria for the diagnosis of osteoporosis in men without fragility fractures have not been firmly established. Although it is clear that low bone mass is a major risk factor for fractures in men, there are insufficient data relating the relative risk of fractures to specific levels of BMD.

Some experts propose that we should use the same criteria as those used in women (T score < − 2.5) and that a normal male reference database should be used to calculate the T scores. Accordingly, men would be diagnosed as having osteoporosis when they are 2.5 standard deviations below peak bone mass for young men but at an absolute BMD that is significantly higher than the absolute BMD at which women are diagnosed. Others argue that we should use the normal female reference database for T-score calculations; in this case, men would be diagnosed

143

as having osteoporosis at the same absolute BMD as women. The estimated prevalence of osteoporosis in men differs, depending on which criteria are used. When the male reference is used, 6% of all men in the U.S. have a T score of < −2.5 at the femoral neck, whereas 4% have a femoral neck T score < −2.5 if the female reference is used. Therefore, use of the male reference will result in significantly more men receiving a diagnosis of osteoporosis and being considered for treatment. It has been further suggested that a T score of −2.5 might not be appropriate and that a male-based T score of approximately −2.0 might be a better diagnostic cut point. Better data comparing the fracture risk for the various proposals and the cost benefit ratios of treatment at each level are clearly indicated. Until such data are available, we recommend the use of a male reference–based T score of −2.5 for the diagnosis of osteoporosis in men.[5–7]

Osteoporosis in men very often occurs as a consequence of another condition or disorder. One large study identified a cause for secondary bone loss in nearly two-thirds of men with osteoporosis, whereas only one-third were thought to have primary (idiopathic) osteoporosis (Fig. 11-1).[8] The more common underlying conditions include hypogonadism, alcohol abuse, glucocorticoid use, and idiopathic hypercalciuria. The use of GnRH analogs to lower serum testosterone levels for the

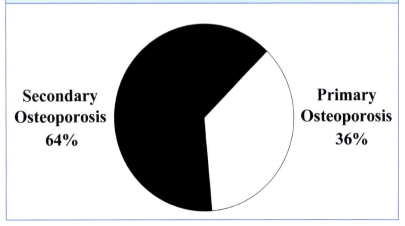

Figure 11-1. Etiology of osteoporosis in men. Approximately 64% of men who have osteoporosis have been reported to have a significant underlying disorder that causes or contributes significantly to their bone loss. The most common disorders identified were hypogonadism, alcohol abuse, glucocorticoid use, and idiopathic hypercalciuria. (Adapted from Kelepouris N, et al: Severe osteoporosis in men. Ann Intern Med 123:452–460, 1995.)

Secondary Osteoporosis 64%

Primary Osteoporosis 36%

treatment of prostate cancer also frequently causes substantial bone loss (Fig. 11-2)[9,10] and increases the risk of fractures in men.[11,12]

The etiology of primary osteoporosis in men, as in women, likely involves a significant genetic component. In addition, testosterone production and serum testosterone levels progressively decline as men age (Fig. 11-3); this is believed to contribute significantly to their age-related development of osteopenia and sarcopenia. However, detailed studies of normal elderly men suggest that testosterone and estrogen are both involved in maintaining bone formation and that estrogen seems to be even more important for the regulation of bone resorption.[13] Supporting this contention, data from the Framingham study indicate that low hip BMD in elderly men is more highly correlated with low serum estradiol levels than with testosterone concentrations.[14]

The evaluation of men with low bone mass or fragility fractures should always include a complete history and physical examination with particular attention to medication use and alcohol consumption, as well as a fall-risk assessment. Laboratory evaluation should consist of measuring serum calcium, phosphorus, creatinine, alkaline phosphatase, and testosterone concentrations; CBC; erythrocyte sedimentation rate; and 24-hour urinary calcium and creatinine excretion. We also recommend lateral thoracic and lumbar spine films to detect any previous vertebral fractures.

Figure 11-2. GnRH analog treatment of prostate cancer reduces BMD in men. In this study, 15 men with prostate cancer were treated with a GnRH analog. As expected, treatment produced highly significant reductions in serum testosterone levels in these men. This was accompanied by significant loss of BMD in the spine, hip, and wrist. (Adapted from Mittan D, et al: Bone loss following hypogonadism in men with prostate cancer treated with GnRH analogs. J Clin Endocrinol Metab 87:3656–3661, 2002.)

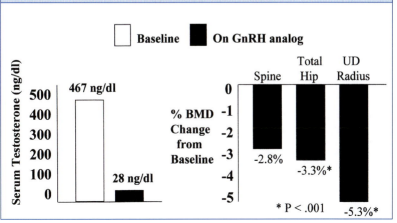

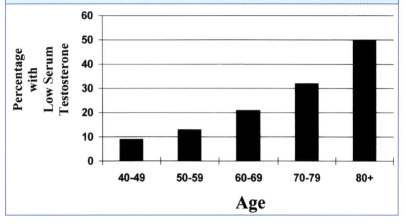

Figure 11-3. Serum testosterone levels in men decline with age. In the Baltimore Longitudinal Study of Aging, serum testosterone levels were measured in 890 men of all ages. The percentage of men with low serum testosterone levels by decade of life increases progressively with age. (Adapted from Harman S, et al: Longitudinal effects of aging on serum total and free testosterone levels in healthy men. Baltimore Longitudinal Study of Aging. J Clin Endocrinol Metab 86:724–731, 2001.)

The treatment of osteoporosis in men consists largely of the same measures used in women. Men should be encouraged to consume a well-balanced diet with adequate amounts of calcium (1500 mg/day) and vitamin D (400 IU/day), to stop smoking, to discontinue or limit alcohol intake, and to exercise regularly (aerobic and resistance exercises). Specific therapy for any identified causes of secondary bone loss should then be instituted. Testosterone replacement, for example, has been shown to significantly increase spinal BMD by as much as 8% in men with frank hypogonadism (low serum testosterone levels) (Fig. 11-4).[15,16] However, it has had insignificant effects in otherwise healthy men who have experienced age-related declines in serum testosterone levels to the low-normal range (Fig. 11-5).[16] Men with idiopathic hypercalciuria can achieve substantial improvements in calcium balance and BMD if they are treated with thiazide diuretics.[17]

Bisphosphonates seem to be as effective in men as they are in women.[18–20] In one study (Fig. 11-6), osteoporotic men given 10 mg of alendronate daily for 2 years exhibited significant BMD increases in the lumbar spine (7.1% vs. baseline; 5.3% vs. placebo), in the femoral neck (2.5% vs. baseline and vs. placebo), and in the total hip (2.0% vs. baseline and vs. placebo).[18] Another study showed a lumbar spine increase of 10.1% (vs. baseline) and a femoral neck increment of 5.2% (vs. baseline) after a 2-year course of daily alendronate.[19] Both studies reported significant reductions of > 50% in the occurrence of new vertebral

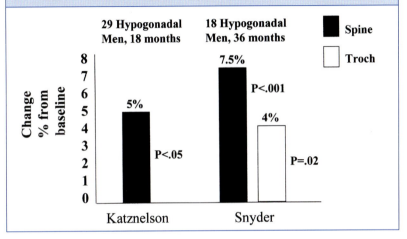

Figure 11-4.   Testosterone replacement increases BMD in hypogonadal men. In two studies, 29 and 18 hypogonadal men were treated with testosterone replacement therapy. BMD increased significantly in response to testosterone replacement in both studies. (Adapted from Katznelson L, et al: Increase in bone density and lean body mass during testosterone administration in men with acquired hypogonadism. J Clin Endocrinol Metab 81:4358–4365, 1996 and Snyder P, et al: Effects of testosterone replacement in hypogonadal men. J Clin Endocrinol Metab 85:2670–2677, 2000.)

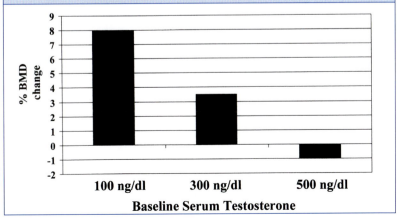

Figure 11-5.   Testosterone replacement increases BMD in men with low serum testosterone levels, but not in those with normal testosterone levels. In this randomized controlled trial, 108 men older than 65 years of age were treated with a testosterone patch or a placebo patch for 36 months. The figure shows changes in BMD for men with normal, low-normal, and frankly low baseline serum testosterone levels. Only those men with frankly low serum testosterone levels had a significant increase in BMD. (Adapted from Snyder P, et al: Effect of testosterone treatment on bone mineral density in men over 65 years of age. J Clin Endocrinol Metab 84:1966–1972, 1999.)

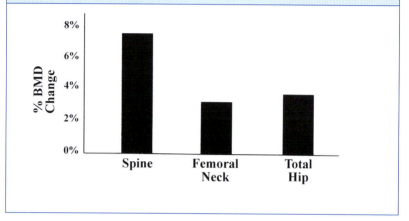

Figure 11-6. **Bisphosphonate therapy increases BMD in men with osteoporosis.** In this randomized controlled trial, 241 men with osteoporosis (age 31–87 years) were given either oral alendronate, 10 mg/day, or a placebo for 2 years. BMD increased 7.1% in the lumbar spine, 2.5% in the femoral neck and 2.0% in the total hip ($P < .001$ compared with baseline and compared with placebo). The incidence of vertebral fractures was reduced by 89% ($P = .02$) in the alendronate group compared with the placebo group. (Adapted from Orwoll E, et al: Alendronate for the treatment of osteoporosis in men. N Engl J Med 343:604–610, 2000.)

fractures. Risedronate has similarly been demonstrated to produce significant 1-year BMD increments in osteoporotic men at the lumbar spine (4.2% vs. baseline; 3.5% vs. placebo), at the femoral neck (1.5% vs. baseline and vs. placebo), and at the total hip (2.3% vs. baseline and vs. placebo).[20] Intravenous pamidronate has been shown to decrease the bone loss associated with GnRH analog use in men with prostate cancer (Fig. 11-7).[21]

Teriparatide (Forteo), a promising new anabolic agent, is under evaluation in a randomized, controlled trial of 437 men. Although the trial was terminated early, preliminary data analysis has revealed significant BMD gains in the spine (5.9% vs. baseline; 5.4% vs. placebo) and in the femoral neck (1.5% vs. baseline; 1.2% vs. placebo) after only 10 months of therapy.[22] The study group also reported a nonsignificant 50% reduction in vertebral fractures (relative risk, 0.50; 95% CI, 0.23–1.12; $P = .086$), but the trial was not adequately powered to accurately assess this end point.[23] Additional research with antiresorptive medications and anabolic agents is ongoing and should provide needed data regarding the optimal approach to the management of osteoporosis in men.

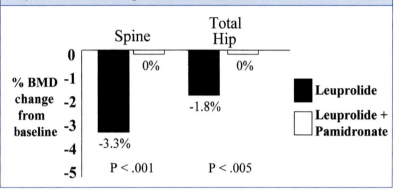

Figure 11-7. Bisphosphonate therapy prevents the loss of BMD resulting from the use of a GnRH analog to treat prostate cancer in men. In this study of 47 men with prostate cancer, treatment with a GnRH analog (Leuprolide) produced significant decrements of BMD, which were completely prevented by the concomitant use of intravenous pamidronate. (Adapted from Smith M, et al: Pamidronate to prevent bone loss during androgen-deprivation therapy for prostatic cancer. N Engl J Med 345:948–955, 2001.)

Key Points: Osteoporosis in Men

- Osteoporosis is a significant disease of men, affecting approximately 1-2 million men in the United States.
- Approximately two-thirds of men with osteoporosis may have a non-skeletal disorder or condition that has contributed significantly to their bone loss.
- The best bone densitometry criteria for making the diagnosis of osteoporosis in men remain controversial. Until more definitive data are available, it is recommended that osteoporosis in men should be defined as a T-score value of −2.5, using a normal male reference population.
- Men with hypogonadism show significant improvement in BMD when they are given testosterone replacement therapy.
- Men respond to antiresorptive and anabolic therapy with increases in BMD that are similar to those seen in women treated with these agents.

References

1. Orwoll ES, Klein RF: Osteoporosis in men. Endocr Rev 16:87–116, 1995.
2. Orwoll ES: Osteoporosis in men. Osteoporosis 27:349–367, 1998.
3. Looker AC, Orwoll ES, Johnston CC Jr, et al: Prevalence of low femoral bone density in older U.S. adults from NHANES III. J Bone Miner Res 12:1761–1768, 1997.

4. Cooper C, Atkinson EJ, Jacobsen SJ, et al: Population-based study of survival after osteoporotic fractures. Am J Epidemiol 137:1001–1005, 1993.
5. Melton III LJ, Atkinson EJ, O'Connor MK, et al: Bone density and fracture risk in men. J Bone Miner Res 13:1915–1923, 1998.
6. Melton III LJ, Orwoll ES, Wasnich RD: Does bone density predict fractures comparably in men and women? Osteoporos Int 12(9):707–709, 2001.
7. Faulkner KG, Orwoll E: Implications in the use of T-scores for the diagnosis of osteoporosis in men. J Clin Densitom 5(1):87–93, 2002.
8. Kelepouris N, Harper KD, Gannon F, et al: Severe osteoporosis in men. Ann Intern Med 123:452–460, 1995.
9. Daniell HW, Dunn SR, Ferguson DW, et al: Progressive osteoporosis during androgen deprivation therapy for prostate cancer. J Urol 163:181–186, 2000.
10. Mittan D, Lee S, Miller E, et al: Bone loss following hypogonadism in men with prostate cancer treated with GnRH analogs. J Clin Endocrinol Metab 87:3656–3661, 2002.
11. Townsend MF, Sanders WH, Northway RO, et al: Bone fractures associated with luteinizing hormone-releasing agonists used in the treatment of prostate carcinoma. Cancer 79:545–550, 1997.
12. Hatano T, Oishi Y, Furuta A, et al: Incidence of bone fracture in patients receiving luteinizing hormone-releasing hormone agonists for prostate cancer. BJU Int 86:449–452, 2000.
13. Falahati-Nini A, Riggs BL, Atkinson EJ, et al: Relative contributions of testosterone and estrogen in regulating bone resorption and formation in normal elderly men. J Clin Invest 106(12):1553–1560, 2000.
14. Amin S, Zhang Y, Sawin CT, et al: Association of hypogonadism and estradiol levels with bone mineral density in elderly men from the Framingham study. Ann Intern Men 133(12):951–963, 2000.
15. Katznelson L, Finkelstein JS, Schoenfeld DA, et al: Increase in bone density and lean body mass during testosterone administration in men with acquired hypogonadism. J Clin Endocrinol Metab 81:4358–4365, 1996.
16. Snyder PJ, Peachey H, Hannoush P, et al: Effect of testosterone treatment on bone mineral density in men over 65 years of age. J Clin Endocrinol Metab 84:1966–1972, 1999.
17. Adams JS, Song CF, Kantorovich V. Rapid recovery of bone mass in hypercalciuric, osteoporotic men treated with hydrochlorothiazide. Ann Intern Med 130(8):658–660, 1999.
18. Orwoll E, Ettinger M, Weiss S, et al: Alendronate for the treatment of osteoporosis in men. N Engl J Med 343:604–610, 2000.
19. Ringe JD, Faber H, Dorst A: Alendronate treatment of established primary osteoporosis in men: results of a 2-year prospective study. J Clin Endocrinol Metab 86:5252–5255, 2001.
20. Ringe JD, Dorst A, Faber H, et al: Risedronate treatment of established primary and secondary osteoporosis in men: 1-year results of a 3-year prospective study. 24th Annual Meeting of the American Society for Bone and Mineral Research, San Antonio, TX, Sept 20–24, 2002, Abstract #SU338.
21. Smith MR, McGovern FJ, Zietman AL, et al: Pamidronate to prevent bone loss during androgen-deprivation therapy for prostate cancer. N Engl J Med 345:948–955, 2001.
22. Orwoll E, Scheele WH, Paul S, et al: The effect of teriparatide [human parathyroid hormone (1-34)] therapy on bone density in men with osteoporosis. J Bone Miner Res 18:9–17, 2003.
23. Orwoll E, Scheele WH, Clancy AD, et al: Recombinant human parathyroid hormone (1-34) therapy reduces the incidence of moderate/severe vertebral fractures in men with low bone density. J Bone Miner Res 16(Suppl. 1):S162, 2001.

Patient Education Materials

Michael McDermott, M.D.
and Carol Zapalowski, M.D., Ph.D.

chapter
12

The following materials may be useful to practitioners who wish to provide educational materials to patients who are interested in preventing, or who need treatment for, osteoporosis. These pamphlets are also available on the following website: www.uchendocrinologypractice.yourmd.com

Osteoporosis Patient Education Pamphlet

1. What is osteoporosis?
Osteoporosis is a common disorder of bones in which they become fragile and likely to fracture easily.
2. What fractures are most commonly associated with osteoporosis?
Fractures of the spine (vertebrae), the hips, and the wrists are most common, but any fracture may occur.
3. What factors contribute most to the risk of a fracture developing?
Low bone mass, age, previous fractures, and an increased tendency to fall down contribute most to the risk of sustaining a fracture.
4. What causes low bone mass?
Risk factors for low bone mass include low calcium intake, low vitamin D intake, lack of exercise, cigarette smoking, drinking excessive alcohol, drinking excessive caffeine, and the use of certain medications such as steroids (prednisone) and excess amounts of thyroid hormone. These conditions can all be corrected.
Risk factors that cannot be changed include age, race (Caucasian, Asian), gender (female), early menopause, slender build, and heredity (family history).
5. How can you know if you have low bone mass?
Bone mass can be measured by a variety of techniques referred to as bone densitometry. Bone densitometry can be used to measure bone mass in your spine, hips, forearms, hands, and heels. Measurement of bone mass at any of these sites can help you estimate your risk of a fracture developing.

6. What conditions make a person more likely to fall?

The use of sedatives, poor vision, Alzheimer's disease, and disabilities of the legs all make an individual more likely to fall down. Falling is also more likely when there are objects in the home over which a person can easily stumble (electrical cords, throw rugs, toys) or conditions that might cause one to slip (slick floors, icy sidewalks).

7. What are the best ways to prevent osteoporosis?

To prevent osteoporosis one should consume an adequate amount of calcium and vitamin D, do regular exercise, stop smoking, limit alcohol intake, limit caffeine consumption, and avoid taking steroids or excess thyroid hormone unless absolutely necessary. Medications such as estrogens, bisphosphonates, and selective estrogen receptor modulators (SERMS) are also good preventive measures. These agents will be discussed later.

8. How do you ensure that you get enough calcium ?

The recommended daily calcium intake is 1000 mg/day in men and premenopausal women and 1500 mg/day in postmenopausal women. The best sources of calcium are dairy products and calcium-fortified citrus juices. Each serving of a dairy product (1 cup of milk, 1 ounce of cheese, 1 cup of yogurt) or calcium-fortified citrus juice (1 cup) has approximately 300 mg of calcium. If you cannot take in enough calcium through your diet, you should take a calcium supplement that adds enough elemental calcium to reach the preceding goals. Calcium carbonate and calcium citrate are two of the most commonly used calcium supplements.

9. How do you ensure that you get enough vitamin D?

The recommended daily vitamin D intake is 400 units. Multivitamins usually contain 400 units per tablet. One or two multivitamin tablets per day will supply all that a person normally needs. More than this should not be taken without medical supervision, because vitamin D can sometimes reach toxic levels in the body if too much is consumed. Other forms of vitamin D are available but should only be prescribed by your health care provider.

10. What types of exercise are best for preventing osteoporosis?

Aerobic exercises such as walking, running, and cycling improve bone mass and strength in the lower spine, hips, and legs. Resistance exercises (weight training) strengthen whatever bones are used during the exercise; these are particularly good for the upper spine and the arms. A combination of aerobic and resistance exercises is more beneficial than either type alone. Exercise also helps to improve balance and coordination and thus reduces the risk of falling. For a specific exercise program that is best for you, you should consult your health-care provider or physical therapist.

11. How much alcohol do you have to drink to harm your bones?

More than two drinks a day seems to increase the risk of osteoporosis.

12. How much caffeine do you have to drink to harm your bones?

More than two servings a day seems to increase the risk of having osteoporosis.

13. Once osteoporosis is present, how can you treat it?

Most of the same measures that are used to prevent osteoporosis are also appropriate treatments for patients who already have osteoporosis. Therefore, individuals with osteoporosis should have an adequate intake of calcium and vitamin D, exercise regularly, stop smoking, limit alcohol and caffeine consumption, and avoid taking steroids or excess doses of thyroid hormone. Medications such as bisphosphonates, estrogens, SERMS, and calcitonin are effective treatment measures for individuals who have osteoporosis.

14. What are bisphosphonates?

Bisphosphonates are a group of medications that prevent bone loss. Currently available bisphosphonates include alendronate (Fosamax), risedronate (Actonel), etidronate (Didronel), and pamidronate (Aredia). Alendronate, risedronate, and etidronate are all oral medications, whereas pamidronate is an intravenously administered preparation. Alendronate and risedronate and are both available in preparations that are taken daily and in preparations that can be taken once a week.

15. How effective are bisphosphonates in preventing and treating osteoporosis?

Bisphosphonates increase bone mass as much as 4%–9% within 2–3 years of starting treatment. Alendronate and risedronate have also been clearly demonstrated to reduce the risk of both vertebral and hip fractures by about 40%–50%.

16. What are the risks and side effects of taking bisphosphonates?

The main side effect of alendronate and risedronate is pain in the lower part of the chest caused by irritation of the esophagus; this occurs in only about 1% of people when the pills are taken properly.

17. What are the instructions for taking Fosamax and Actonel properly?

Fosamax and Actonel should be taken first thing in the morning with a full glass of water. The person should then remain upright and take nothing else by mouth (food, drink, or medications) for 30–60 minutes afterwards. These measures serve to minimize the risk of side effects and to maximize the absorption of the medication from the intestine into the bloodstream.

18. What types of estrogens are available for hormone replacement therapy?

Commonly used oral estrogen preparations include conjugated estrogens (Premarin, Ogen, Cenestin), esterified estrogens (Menest), estropipate (Ortho-Est), estradiol (Estrace, Estradiol), and combinations of estrogen with progesterone (PremPro, PremPhase, Ortho-Prefest, FemHRT, Activella). Estrogen skin patches (Estraderm, Vivelle, Climara, Alora, Esclim) and combination estrogen/progesterone patches (Combipatches) are preferred for some individuals.

19. How effective are estrogens in the prevention and treatment of osteoporosis?

Estrogen replacement therapy prevents postmenopausal bone loss. When started near the time of menopause, estrogens increase bone mass by about 4%. They have similar effects when given to women with established osteoporosis, even those women who are more than 15 years past menopause. Estrogens combined with progesterone were shown in the Women's Health Initiative (WHI) study to reduce the risk of both vertebral and hip fractures by approximately 34%.

20. What other benefits result from taking estrogens?

Estrogen replacement therapy reduces postmenopausal hot flashes, genital atrophy, and probably depression. In the WHI study, estrogens were shown to reduce the risk of colon cancer moderately. Some reports suggest that estrogens may also decrease the risk of Alzheimer's disease.

21. What are the risks and side effects of taking estrogens?

Estrogen replacement therapy increases the risk of having cancer of the endometrium (lining of the uterus); taking progesterone with estrogens effectively prevents this complication. Estrogens also modestly increase the risk of breast cancer. In addition, estrogens increase the risk of blood clots in the legs and pelvis; these clots can sometimes break loose and go to the lungs. All these complications are more likely to occur with higher doses of estrogen. In the WHI study, estrogens given with progesterone were found to moderately increase the risk of heart attacks.

22. What are plant estrogens or phytoestrogens?

Phytoestrogens are estrogen-like substances found in a variety of plants. There have been approximately 20 such substances identified in nearly 300 different types of plants, including soybeans, parsley, garlic, wheat, rice, dates, pomegranates, cherries, coffee, and many herbs. The three main classes of phytoestrogens are the isoflavanoids, the coumestans, and the lignans. The best studied are the isoflavanoids (genistein, daidzein), which are found in soy-based foods. In humans, these compounds have weak estrogen activity compared with conjugated estrogens and estradiol.

The effects of phytoestrogens on bone mass are not well studied, but there is some evidence that they may prevent or diminish bone loss in women after menopause. They have not, however, been shown to reduce the risk of fractures. Although phytoestrogens may seem to be an attractive alternative to estrogen therapy in women who do not wish to take estrogens, they cannot, at this time, be considered proven measures for the prevention and treatment of osteoporosis.

23. What are SERMS?

These medications mimic estrogen actions in some of the body's tissues (e.g., bones) and inhibit normal estrogen actions in other tissues (e.g., breast). Currently available SERMS include raloxifene (Evista) and tamoxifen (Nolvadex).

24. How effective are SERMS in the prevention and treatment of osteoporosis?

Raloxifene increases bone mass by about 2%–3% in postmenopausal women and reduces the risk of vertebral fractures by about 40%–50%.

25. Are there other benefits to taking SERMS?

Raloxifene and tamoxifen have been shown to reduce the risk of breast cancer.

26. What are the risks and side effects of taking SERMS?

These medications can cause hot flashes and, like estrogens, may increase the risk of blood clots in the legs and pelvis.

27. What is calcitonin?

Calcitonin is a natural hormone produced in the thyroid gland; it prevents bone loss. Calcitonin is available as a nasal spray (Miacalcin) and as an injectable liquid (Miacalcin and Calcimar).

28. How effective is calcitonin in preventing and treating osteoporosis?

The administration of calcitonin to patients with osteoporosis increases bone mass minimally but reduces the risk of vertebral fracture by about 33%. Calcitonin also has some analgesic properties, reducing back pain in approximately 80% of treated patients.

29. What are the risks and side effects of taking calcitonin?

Calcitonin administration may cause nausea and a skin rash. Nasal spray calcitonin may also cause irritation of the inside of the nose.

30. What is teriparatide (Forteo)?

Teriparatide (Forteo) is a shortened form of parathyroid hormone (PTH), which is a natural hormone made by the parathyroid glands, located in the neck next to the thyroid gland. PTH is the body's most important regulator of calcium metabolism. When given as an injection once a day, Forteo stimulates new bone formation.

31. How effective is Forteo for the treatment of osteoporosis?

Treating patients with Forteo for 18 months increases bone mass by about 10%–14% in the spine and by 3%–5% in the hip. It also reduces the risk of fractures in the spine by 65%–70%. Forteo must be given as a daily injection (shot).

32. Is it useful to combine these medications?

Combinations of a bisphosphonate (Fosamax or Actonel) with either estrogens or Evista have been shown to increase bone mass more than single drugs used alone. Combination therapy is therefore commonly used in people with severe osteoporosis. Estrogens should not be used with Evista, however, because these two medications have opposing actions.

33. Are male hormones, like testosterone, beneficial for women with osteoporosis?

Small amounts of testosterone given along with estrogen seem to improve bone mass more than does estrogen treatment alone. This may also improve libido (sex drive). However, side effects can include facial hair growth, deepening of the voice, and decreases in the blood level of HDL cholesterol (the good type). The use of the lowest doses of testosterone possible can minimize or prevent these side effects. DHEA is also currently under study.

34. What other medications may be useful in treating osteoporosis?

Slow-release sodium fluoride and growth hormone are under study as possible treatments for osteoporosis. These medications increase bone mass significantly, but their long-term safety and their ability to prevent bone fractures must be demonstrated before they can be approved for general use.

35. How is osteoporosis treated in men?

Men with osteoporosis should consume adequate intakes of calcium and vitamin D, should exercise regularly, should stop smoking, and should minimize alcohol and caffeine consumption. Osteoporosis in men often results from an underlying medical disorder. These conditions should be identified and treated appropriately. For example, men who have low serum testosterone levels should be treated with testosterone replacement therapy. Bisphosphonates (Fosamax, Actonel) seem to be as effective in men with osteoporosis as they are in women (see earlier).

36. Why do steroid medications cause osteoporosis?

Steroid medications, given in moderate to high doses (prednisone doses > 7 mg/day) increase bone loss and impair new bone formation. Osteoporosis can appear within 6 months of starting treatment with these medications. These medications are generally used for inflammatory conditions of the joints, lungs, intestines, kidneys, and skin. They are also used, along with other medications, in people who have had organ transplantations.

37. How can osteoporosis from steroid medications be prevented and treated?

All people who take steroids should consume 1500 mg of calcium and 800 units of vitamin D (2 multivitamins) each day and should exercise regularly, stop smoking, and minimize alcohol and caffeine consumption. People who will be on steroid medications for 3 months or more should be considered for additional treatment with bisphosphonates (Fosamax, Actonel), estrogens, or calcitonin.

Content of Calcium Supplements

Contents of Some Brand-Name Calcium Preparations		
Preparation	**Elemental Calcium per Tablet in (milligrams)**	**Vitamin D in Preparations Supplemented with Vitamin D* (in IU per tablet)**
Calcium carbonate		
Caltrate	600 mg	200 IU
Oscal	500 mg	200 IU
Viactiv	500 mg	100 IU
Tums**	200 mg	0 IU
Tums EX**	300 mg	0 IU
Tums Ultra**	400 mg	0 IU
Tums 500**	500 mg	0 IU
Nature Made	500 mg	200 IU
Nature Made	600 mg	200 IU
Maalox†	222 mg	0 IU
Rolaids†	250 mg	0 IU
Calcium citrate		
Citracal‡	200 mg	0 IU
Citracal‡	250 mg	62.5 IU
Citracal‡	315 mg	200 IU
Multiple vitamins		
Women's One-a-Day	450 mg	400 IU
Centrum Silver	200 mg	400 IU

*Many calcium supplements are formulated as preparations with vitamin D and without vitamin D.
**On the Tums bottles, both the full weight of two pills and a table with mg of elemental calcium for two tablets are shown. For example, Tums EX is listed as 600 mg of elemental calcium for two tablets with the total weight of 810 mg of calcium carbonate in two pills.
†Both Maalox and Rolaids are listed as the full weight of calcium carbonate in two tablets on the outside label. For Maalox, the full weight of one tablet is listed as 600 mg, and for Rolaids, the full weight of the one tablet is listed as 675 mg.
‡All the Citracal preparations are listed as the amount for two pills on the label.

Exercises for Improving Bone Strength and Body Balance

Beginning Exercise Program

1. Toe raises
   a. Stand flatfooted facing a wall or doorjamb
   b. Place hands on hips, or
   c. Place hand on the wall or doorjamb for balance, if needed
   d. Rise to the balls of your feet; then return to the floor
   e. Start: 2 sets of 5 repetitions each
   f. Goal: 3 sets of 15 repetitions each

2. Chair stands
   a. Sit upright in a chair
   b. Hold arms directly in front of you, or
   c. Hold armrests for balance, if needed
   d. Rise to a standing position; then return to seat
   e. Goal: 3 sets of 25 repetitions each
3. Standing hip flexion
   a. Stand flatfooted next to a wall or doorjamb
   b. Place hands on hips, or
   c. Place hand on the wall or doorjamb for balance, if needed
   d. Raise right knee to hip level with knee bent; return to floor
   e. Goal: 3 sets of 25 repetitions on each side
4. Horizontal trunk raises (modified crunches)
   a. Lie flat on floor or bed with knees bent at 90-degree angle
   b. Hold arms across chest or behind head
   c. Raise shoulders up 6–12 inches; then lie back down
   d. Goal: 3 sets of 25 repetitions each
5. Shoulder shrugs
   a. Stand upright
   b. Keep hands down at your sides
   c. Hold a 5-lb. dumbbell in each hand
   d. Shrug shoulders straight up; then return to start position
   e. Goal: 3 sets of 20 repetitions each
6. Upward arm presses (military press)
   a. Stand upright
   b. Hold your hands, palms forward, in front of your shoulders
   c. Hold a 5-lb. dumbbell in each hand
   d. Push hands straight up, all the way; then return to start position
   e. Goal: 3 sets of 20 repetitions each
7. Walk 45 minutes each day, 6 days a week

Educational Websites of Interest

appendix

The National Osteoporosis Foundation
   www.nof.org
NIH Osteoporosis and Related Bone Diseases–National Resource Center
   www.osteo.org
American Society for Bone and Mineral Research
   www.asbmr.org
Bones and Osteoporosis
   www.bones-and-osteoporosis.com
Osteoporosis Continuing Medical Education
   www.osteoporosiscme.org
West Central Regional Osteoporosis Board
   www.wcrob.org
The Endocrine Society
   www.endo-society.org
The American Association of Clinical Endocrinologists
   www.aace.com
The Hormone Foundation
   www.hormone.org
The American College of Obstetrics and Gynecology
   www.acog.org
The North American Menopause Society
   www.menopause.org
The Endocrine Practice, University of Colorado Hospital
   www.uchendocrinologypractice.yourmd.com